NUTRIENTS AS ERGOGENIC AIDS FOR SPORTS AND EXERCISE

T0186445

Luke Bucci, Ph.D., C.C.N., C(A.S.C.P.)
Director
InnerPath Nutrition
Houston, Texas

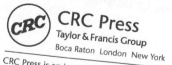

CRC Press
Taylor & Francis Group
Boca Raton London New York

CRC Press is an imprint of the
Taylor & Francis Group, an **informa** business

CRC Press
Taylor & Francis Group
6000 Broken Sound Parkway NW, Suite 300
Boca Raton, FL 33487-2742

© 1993 by Taylor & Francis Group, LLC
CRC Press is an imprint of Taylor & Francis Group, an Informa business

First issued in paperback 2019

No claim to original U.S. Government works

ISBN 13: 978-0-367-45004-5 (pbk)
ISBN 13: 978-0-8493-4223-3 (hbk)

Library of Congress Cataloging-in-Publication Data

Bucci, Luke R.
    Nutrients as ergogenic aids for sports and exercise / Luke R. Bucci.
        p.   cm. – (Nutrition in exercise and sport)
    Includes bibliographical references and index.
    ISBN 0-8493-4223-6
        1. Energy metabolism. 2. Dietary supplements. 3. Exercise–Physiological
    aspects. I. Title. II. Series.
        [DNLM: 1. Amino Acids. 2. Energy Metabolism. 3. Exertion–drug effects. 4. Food,
    Fortified. 5. Minerals. 6. Vitamins. QT 135 B918n]
    QP176.B83 1993
    613.2'08'8796—dc20
    DNLM/DLC
                                                                            92-49997
                                                                            CIP

Library of Congress Card Number 92-49997

AUTHOR

Luke R. Bucci, Ph.D., C.C.N., C(A.S.C.P.), is Director of Science and Quality for SpectraCell Laboratories, Inc., a clinical testing facility that examines nutritional and metabolic functions by *in vitro* culture of lymphocytes in a series of specially designed media. Dr. Bucci is also Director of InnerPath Nutrition, a nutritional consulting and educational enterprise.

Dr. Bucci received his B.Sc. in Chemistry from St. Edward's University, Austin, Texas, in 1977. The Graduate School of Biomedical Sciences, University of Texas Health Science Center at Houston, granted him a Ph.D. in Biomedical Sciences in 1983. While engaged in graduate work, Dr. Bucci received Rosalie B. Hite Memorial Fellowships, as well as the Rosalie B. Hite Memorial Merit Award for Outstanding Research in 1983. His dissertation topic was concerned with changes in cell nuclear proteins during spermatogenesis.

An appointment followed as Project Investigator for the Department of Experimental Radiotherapy, University of Texas System Cancer Center, M.D. Anderson Hospital, in Houston, Texas, where effects of chemotherapy and radiation therapies on normal animal and human tissues were studied. Dr. Bucci became Director of Research for Biotics Research Corporation in Houston, Texas, and a Technical Advisor for Sports Research Corporation in 1984. These companies manufactured nutritional supplements for health care practitioners and the retail sports market, respectively. Dr. Bucci continued to research ergogenic aids and to deliver educational seminars on sports nutrition until 1991, when InnerPath Nutrition was formed. In addition, Dr. Bucci received a certification as a clinical nutritionist (C.C.N.) from the International and American Associations of Clinical Nutritionists (IAACN). He is currently a member of the Board of Trustees for the Clinical Nutrition Certification Board of the IAACN. Dr. Bucci is also a Technologist in Chemistry certified by the American Society of Clinical Pathology.

AUTHOR

Luke R. Bucci, Ph.D., C.C.N., C.(A.S.C.P.) is Director of Science and Quality for SpectraCell Laboratories, Inc., a clinical testing facility that examines nutritional and metabolic functions by in vitro culture of lymphocytes in a series of specially designed media. Dr. Bucci is also Director of InterHealth Nutrition, a nutritional consulting and educational enterprise.

Dr. Bucci received his B.Sc. in Chemistry from St. Edward's University, Austin, Texas, in 1977. The Graduate School of Biomedical Sciences, University of Texas Health Science Center at Houston, granted him a Ph.D. in Biomedical Sciences in 1984. While engaged in graduate work, Dr. Bucci received Rosalie B. Hite Memorial Fellowships, as well as the Rosalie B. Hite Memorial Merit Award for Outstanding Research in 1981. His dissertation topic was concerned with changes in cell nuclear proteins during spermatogenesis.

An appointment followed as Project Investigator for the Department of Experimental Radiotherapy, University of Texas System Cancer Center, M.D. Anderson Hospital in Houston, Texas, where effects of chemotherapy and radiation therapies on normal animal and human tissues were studied. Dr. Bucci became Director of Research for Biotics Research Corporation in Houston, Texas, and a Technical Advisor for Sports Research Corporation in 1984. These companies manufactured nutritional supplements for health care practitioners and the retail sports market, respectively. Dr. Bucci continued to research, suggesting aids and to deliver educational seminars on sports nutrition until 1991, when InterHealth Nutrition was formed. In addition, Dr. Bucci received a certification as a clinical nutritionist (C.C.N.) from the International and American Associations of Clinical Nutritionists (IAACN). He is currently a member of the Board of Trustees for the Clinical Nutrition Certification Board of the IAACN. Dr. Bucci is also a Technologist in Chemistry certified by the American Society of Clinical Pathology.

PREFACE

The CRC Series Nutrition in Exercise and Sport is designed to provide the setting for indepth exploration of the many and varied aspects of nutrition and exercise, including sport. The topic of sports nutrition gained real interest among physiologists in the 1960s and since then numerous scientific studies have been performed, many of which have focused on healthful benefits of good nutrition and exercise. As we enter the present decade and move forward, scientists will search ever more elusive "optimum" nutritional preparation. As they try to unlock nature's secrets, it will be necessary to remember that there must be a range of diets that will support excellent physical performance. Yet, there will inevitably be attempts by scientists and laymen alike to distill the diets to some common denominator — a formula for success. The CRC Series on Nutrition in Exercise and Sport is dedicated to providing a stage to explore these issues. Each volume seeks to provide a detailed and scholarly examination of some aspect of the topic. Ultimately, the series will comprise a set of authoritative volumes for consultation by scientists, physicians, and a broad range of healthcare providers and individuals who participate in exercise and sport, whether for recreation or competition.

We welcome the contribution by Luke Bucci, *Nutrients as Ergogenic Aids for Sports and Exercise,* to the series. (Due to the rapid expansion of research on sports nutrition, sections updated during production have reference numbers out of sequence from the rest of the text.)

James F. Hickson, Jr., Ph.D., R.D.
Ira Wolinsky, Ph.D.
Series Editors

FOREWORD

Ergogenesis is the production of energy. Ergogenic aids are nutrients used to improve energy production, and thus, human performance. The enhancement of human performance by nutritional means has been studied and applied for thousands of years. Until this century, only foodstuffs could be manipulated in an effort to improve performance. Presently, the ability to provide almost any nutrient or cellular compound in sufficient quantity to market, coupled with a better understanding of human metabolism and exercise physiology, has resulted in an explosion of ideas and products with specific applications to exercising people. While much research has been performed, and many basic questions about nutrition and exercise have been answered, many more questions remain. This gap between what is hypothetical and what is known has been filled by a plethora of sophisticated products which have received little if any rigorous scientific examination for efficacy. Nevertheless, sports nutrition is big business, attracting attention from a wide variety of suppliers, ranging from pharmaceutical and food industry conglomerates to "mom and pop" operations.

This author has personal experience with both rigorous, academic scientific examination of nutrients as ergogenic aids, as well as commercial application of nutritional supplements from an industrial and clinical viewpoint. Certain observations about the reality of nutritional ergogenic aids have become apparent. A segment of our society is convinced that certain "foods" (for example, desiccated liver tablets) can produce decisive results in physical training. These convictions are based on no firm scientific observations. Obscure citations on physiological effects of a particular compound have been used to create and promote healthy sales of that compound, without proof from actual applied research. Anecdotal comments by successful sportsmen have been turned into nutritional dogma through word of mouth. Peer-reviewed scientific journal articles have been misinterpreted, misquoted, misunderstood, and misused to promote products. People are obviously willing to invest in any edge that will improve performance. This desire is central to success in athletics and training, and it is to be commended.

On the other hand, preconceived biases on the part of some academic investigators have led to the publication of time-consuming and expensive research studies that were doomed from the start to fail in finding any ergogenic effects. If one supplements nutrients at doses well known to be insufficient to change the way the body handles those nutrients, then one can expect no changes in physiological, biochemical, or performance measurements. Sweeping conclusions on the ineffectiveness of ergogenic aids in general are not based on firm scientific grounds.

Fortunately, most researchers are objective enough to design and implement rational studies, and from these results, a large body of literature has actually found that dietary manipulations, under the proper settings, can indeed benefit exercise performance. Of course, many studies have shown the futility of using some nutrients as ergogenic aids. That any conclusions at all can be derived from studies that endeavor to decipher the overwhelmingly entangled interactions among nutrition, metabolism, and sports is a tribute to the keen minds of researchers in the field of exercise physiology and sports nutrition.

If the knowledge base of nutritional ergogenic aids can be imagined as a continuum from 0 to 100%, I believe we have arrived at 55%. This book was written to offer a slightly different perspective on nutrients as ergogenic aids to human exercise performance in order to further the knowledge score of the continuum. Topics, such as amino acids, not normally considered or discussed in scientific studies are addressed in a rational manner, with the hope that further applied research can be stimulated. Regardless of whether actual published results of studies exist or not, these compounds and many others have been in practical use by thousands of people for over a dozen years. Thus, researchers are forced into a catch-up situation with respect to influencing the opinions of users. Many users of nutritional ergogenic aids maintain that they *feel* a difference when these compounds are consumed, fostering their continued use. It is difficult to argue with the feelings of others.

This book is concerned primarily with results from human studies, with minimal reliance on animal data. Interaction of exercise with nutrition has not been examined, in order to maintain the focus on the application of nutrients to enhance performance. Relevance to real-life situations is considered, and whenever possible, guidelines on safe use are presented. The reader is urged to examine carefully the applicability of these guidelines for his/her individual purposes. In order to spur interest in applied research, even speculative guidelines are presented. This is not to condone benefits, but to suggest guidelines for the more adventurous.

Only with more knowledge can truth be illuminated. It is hoped that this book will become another step to bridge the gap between cult and science, stimulating further research and sensible applications of nutrient modulation to benefit exercise performance.

Luke R. Bucci, Ph.D., C.C.N., C(A.S.C.P.)
June, 1992

ACKNOWLEDGMENTS

Assistance from the U.S. Olympic Committee, R. O. Voy, M.D., and his staff is gratefully acknowledged, as is permission to reproduce their hotline telephone number. Naniece Bucci and Rose Kelly deserve praise for their excellent handling of the manuscript. This book is dedicated to the memory of Michael Kazilas.

TABLE OF CONTENTS

INTRODUCTION

I. DEFINITIONS AND HISTORICAL BACKGROUND

Ergogenic aids are substances or devices used to improve exercise and athletic performance by improving the production of energy. Athletic events are competitive by nature, and any boost in performance, no matter how trivial, is desired and pursued vigorously by athletes and coaches. Anything that can be imagined or perceived to aid some aspect of performance has probably been tried in a ceaseless quest for a margin of victory. Perhaps the grandfather of those who have used ergogenic aids is Dromeus of Stymphalus, who, in 450 B.C., espoused ingestion of muscle meat to improve muscular strength.[1] Aztec warriors ate the hearts of particularly brave adversaries in an attempt to gain that bravery. Later, practices such as water deprivation, purging of body toxins by bloodletting, leeching, vomiting, or use of enemas, and ingestion of unusual dietary items became commonplace.[2] With advances in science and technology, numerous substances and devices have been applied to the improvement of human performance. The disciplines of nutrition, biochemistry, pharmacology, and exercise physiology have accumulated a large body of data, albeit incomplete, concerning the effects of exogenous aids on exercise performance.

This book will briefly present some findings on nonnutritional ergogenic aids and then will focus on available information on nutritional ergogenic aids. Nutritional ergogenic aids are defined as dietary components that are ingested in order to enhance or improve exercise and/or sports performance. Nutritional ergogenic aids can be foodstuffs and their components, such as pasta or starch, or even compounds better known as metabolic intermediates, such as coenzyme Q_{10}. Also included are some components of plants that are familiar (caffeine) or still obscure (ferulates). When applicable, practical guidelines will be given on when and how to use nutritional ergogenic aids.

Chapter 1

NONNUTRITIONAL ERGOGENIC AIDS

I. INTRODUCTION

Ergogenic aids may be grouped into several categories: mechanical, psychological, physiological, pharmacological, and nutritional. Table 1 lists some of the more popular mechanical, psychological, and physiological aids. Reviews by Brooks and Fahey,[3] deVries,[4] Karpovich,[5] McArdle, et al.,[6] Morgan,[7] and Williams[8] explore postulated mechanisms and research results on these aids.

II. PHARMACOLOGICAL AIDS

A. RELATION OF DRUGS TO NUTRITION

Pharmacological aids deserve special mention because of their widespread use and close relation to nutritional aids. Most pharmacological aids are prescription drugs, including synthetic compounds and nature-identical substances. Use of nonprescription drugs offers a real threat of suspension from athletic activities if the athlete consumes certain compounds inadvertently. Sometimes, pharmaceutical products contain both nutrients and drugs. Also, drugs may have significant effects on performance due to alterations of nutritional status. Thus, the relationship between certain pharmaceutical agents and nutrition will be reviewed briefly.

Table 2 presents a brief list of drug categories and effects related to nutrition. It is beyond the scope of this chapter to fully explore interactions between drugs and nutritional status. However, possible effects of drugs on nutritional status may have a negative impact upon performance by depleting fuels, water, electrolytes, or essential micronutrients.[9] Likewise, some drugs may enhance performance by causing dietary changes in food consumption.[9]

III. FOODSTUFFS AS BANNED SUBSTANCES

Another concern is the identification of naturally-occurring compounds in certain herbs which are not commonly considered as substances banned for athletic competition. Examples include caffeine in guarana, coffee, tea, and "energy" nutritional supplements or ephedrines in Ma Huang (Chinese Ephedra). Consumption of large amounts of dietary supplements containing these herbs may result in a positive drug test when U.S. Olympic Committee (USOC) drug testing methods are used, which then could lead to accidental disbarment at athletic events. While it is difficult to predict accurately just how much of an herbal product will cause illegal levels of banned substances, the following

TABLE 1
Some Nonnutritional Ergogenic Aids in Current Practice

Mechanical	Psychological	Physiological
Body hair removal	Biofeedback	Biorhythm timing
Braces	Hypnosis	Blood reinfusion
Gait analysis	Meditation	Colonics/Enemas
Occlusal splints	Music	Electrical
Orthotic devices	Mental imaging	Stimulation
Shoe designs	Placebos	Manipulation
Streamlined	Pep talks	Massage
Clothes/helmets	Social factors	Negatively ionized
	Stress reduction	air
	Subliminal tapes	Pure oxygen
	Superstitions	breathing
		Polarization
		Sunlight/colors
		Warm-up
		Yoga

Note   This table is intended as a list of some ergogenic aids in current use, and it does not necessarily condone efficacy.

TABLE 2
Interaction of Pharmaceuticals with Nutrition

Drug category	Nutritional relationships
Anabolic/Androgenic steroids	Increased appetite
	Decreased catabolism
	Altered lipoprotein levels
	Reduced high-density cholesterol levels
Antihistamines	Decreased appetite
Amphetamines	Decreased appetite
	Increased metabolic rate
Diuretics	Dehydration and electrolyte loss
Oral contraceptives	Altered handling of micronutrients
Corticosteroids	Increased catabolism (muscle wasting)
	Altered metabolism of essential nutrients
Thyroid hormones	Increased metabolic rate
Somatotropin (growth hormone)	Hypoglycemia
Insulin	Hypoglycemia

crude guidelines may be used: (1) caffeine — more than five to six cups of fresh-brewed coffee or more than five to six caffeine tablets; (2) ephedrine — any amount of over-the-counter decongestant or herbal product containing Ma Huang (Chinese Ephedra). The ergogenic effects of these compounds found in foodstuffs will be examined later in this section.

Likewise, increasing abuse of hormones identical to those found in the human body may affect levels of nutrients.[10,11] Somatotropin (human growth hormone), erythropoietin, insulin, and thyroxine (T4) are some examples.

IV. BANNED PHARMACOLOGICAL SUBSTANCES

Table 3 is a partial list of the substances banned by the USOC.[12] An athlete or coach is strongly encouraged to consult the toll-free Drug Information Hotline of the USOC (800-233-0393) before an athlete consumes any medication or unusual dietary aid prior to a competitive event.

Further information on the effects of pharmaceuticals on performance may be found in the reviews by Brooks and Fahey,[3] Goldman,[13] Haupt,[14] Wagner,[11] and Williams.[8,9]

A. ANABOLIC STEROIDS

Anabolic steroids deserve separate mention owing to their epidemic use and possible nutritional demands on users. Specific reviews on results and side effects are presented by Haupt and Rovere,[15] Hickson, et al.,[16] Kochakian,[17] Kibble and Ross,[18] Kleiner,[19] Kruskemper,[20] Wright,[21] and the National Strength and Conditioning Association (NSCA).[22] As mentioned previously, anabolic steroids lead to increases in appetite. In addition, a critical review of 24 studies on subjects using anabolic steroids found a possible association between high protein diets and strength increases.[15] However, conclusive evidence is still lacking that protein supplements or high-protein diets (in excess of 2 g/kg/d) enhance or hasten the effects of anabolic steroids. Anabolic steroid users continue to consume high dietary levels of protein, sometimes with concomitant high-fat intake, which may increase the risk of cardiovascular disease, as anabolic steroids increase low density lipoprotein levels and dramatically reduce high density lipoprotein levels.[23–29] Dietary manipulation studies to modify lipoprotein levels in steroid users are still lacking.

TABLE 3
Drugs Banned by the USOC

Alcohol
Prohibited in certain instances

Anabolic steroids
Bolasterone
Boldenone (Vebonol™)
Clostebol (Steranobol™)
Danazol (Danocrine™)
Ethylestrenol (Maxibolin™)
Fluoxymesterone (Android F. Halotestin)
Mesterolone (Androviron™, Proviron™)
Methandrostenolone (Dianabol™, Andoredan™)
Methenolone (Primobolan™, Primabolan-Depot™)
Methyltestosterone (Android™, Estratest™, Methandren™, Oreton™, Testred™)
    nandrolone (Durabolin™, Deca-Durabolin™, Kabolin™, Nandrobolic™)
Norenthandrolone (Nilevar™)
Oxandrolone (Anavar™, Antitriol™)
Oxymesterone (Oranabol™, Theranabol™)
Oxymetholone (Anadrol™, Nilevar™, Anapolon 50™, Adroyd™)
Stanozolol (Winstrol™, Stromba™)
Testosterones and derivatives (Maolgen™, Malogex™, Delatestryl™, Oreton™)

Human growth hormone (not a steroid, but considered an anabolic)
Growth hormone releasing hormone (not a steroid, but considered an anabolic)

Beta-blockers
Acebutolol (Sectral™)
Labetalol (Normodyne™, Trandate™)
Metoprolol (Lopressor™)
Nadolol (Corgard™)
Oxprenolol (Apsolox™, Oxanol™, Transacor™)
Pindolol (Visken™)
Propanolol (Inderal™)
Timolol (Blocarden™)

Corticosteroids
The use of corticosteroids is banned except for topical use (aural, opthamological, and
    dermatological), inhalational therapy (asthma, allergic rhinitis), and local or
    intraarticular injection
Any team doctor wishing to administer corticosteroids intraarticularly or locally to a
    competitor must give written notification to the International Olympic Committee
    (IOC) medical commission.

Diuretics
Acetazolamide (Diamox™, Dazamide™)
Amiloride (Midamor™)
Bendroflumethazide (Naturetin™)
Benzthiazide (Aquatag™, Exna™, Hydrex™, Marazide™, Proaqua™)
Bumetanide (Bumex™)
Chlortalidone (Hygroton™, Hylidone™, Thalitone™)

TABLE 3 (continued)
Drugs Banned by the USOC

Diclofenamide (Daranide™)
Ethacrynic acid (Edecrin™)
Furosemide (Lasix™)
Hydrochlorothiazide (Esidrex™, Hydrodiuril™, Oretic™, Thiuretid™)
Spironolactone (Alatone™, Aldactone™)
Triamterene (Dyrenium™, Dyazide™)

Local anesthetics
  Only local or intraarticular injections when medically justified (procaine, xylocaine, carbocaine)

Narcotics and analgesics
  Buprenorphine (Buprenex™)
  Codeine (Tylenol-III™, Codicept™)
  Diamorphine (Heroin™)
  Dihydrocodeine (Synalgos DC™, Paracodin™)
  Ethlymorphine (Dionin™)
  Hydrocodone (Hycodan™, Tussionex™)
  Hydromorphone (Dilaudid™)
  Methadone (Amidon™, Dolophine™)
  Morphine (Duromorph™, Cyclimorph 10™)
  Oxocodone (Percodan™, Vicodan™)
  Oxomorphine (Narcan™)
  Pethidine (Demerol™, Centralgin™, Colantin™)
  Phenazocine (Narphen™, Primadol™)
  Tincture opium (Paregoric™)
  Trimeperidine (Demerol™, Mepergan™)

Stimulants
  Amfepramone (Apisate™, Tenuate™, Tenpanil™)
  Amiphenazole (Dapti™, Daptizole™, Amphisol™)
  Amphetamine (Delcobese™, Obetrol™, Benzedrine™, Dexedrine™)
  Benzphetamine (Didrex™)
  Caffeine[a]
  Cocaine (Surfacaine™, coke, snow, crack, etc)
  Diethylproprion (Tenuate™, Tepanil™)
  Dimetamfetamine (Amphetamine)
  Ephedrine (Bronkaid™, Bronkotabs™, Collyrium™, Ma Huang™ or Chinese Ephedra™, Nyquil™ Nighttime Cold Medicine, Pazo™ Suppository, Primatene™, Rynatuss™, Tedral™, Vicks™ Nighttime Cold Medicine, Vitronol™ Nose Drops, Wyanoid™ Suppository)
  Etafedrine (Mercodal™, Decapryn™, Metamine™)
  Fencamfamine (Envitrol™, Altimine™, Phencamine™)
  Isoetharine (Bronkosol™, Bronkometer™, Numotac™, Dilabron™)
  Isoproterenol (Isuprel™, Norisodrine™, Metihaler™, Iso™)
  Meclofenoxate (Lucidril™, Brenal™)
  Mefenorex (Doracil™, Pondinil™, Rondimen™)
  Methamphetamine (Desoxyn™, Met-Ampi™)
  Methoxyphenamine (Ritalin™, Orthoxicol™)
  Methylephedrine (Tzbraine™, Methep™)

TABLE 3 (continued)
Drugs Banned by the USOC

Methylphenidate (Ritalin™)
Nikethamide (Coramine™)
Norpseudoephedrine
Pemolin (Cylert™, Deltamin™, Stimul™)
Phendimetrazine (Phenazine™, Bontril™, Plegine™)
Phenmetrazine (Preludin™)
Phenylephrine (Corocidin™, Dristan™, NTZ™, Neo-Synephrine™, Sinex™)
Phenylpropanolamine (Arm™, Allerest™, Contact™, Dexatrim™, Dietac™, 4-way
    Formula 44™, Naldecon™, Novahistine™, Sine-Aid™, Sine-Off™, Sinutab™,
    Triaminic™, Triaminicin™, Sucrets™ Cold Decongestant, many related products)
Propylhexedrine (Benzedrex™ Inhaler)
Pseudoephedrine (Actifed™, Ambenyl™, Anamine™, Afrinol™, Co-Tylenol™,
    Deconamine™, Dicamol™, Emprazil™, Fedahist™, Fedrazil™, Histalet™, Historal™,
    Isoclor™, Lo-Tussin™, Nasalspan™, Novafed™, Nucofed™, Poly-Hisine™, Pseudo-
    Bid™, Pseudo-Hist™, Rhymosyn™, Ryne™, Sudafed™, Triprolidine™, Tussend™,
    Chlorafed™, Chlortrimetron-DC™, Disophoral™, Drixoral™, Polaramine™, Rondec™)
Strychnine (Movellan™)

Permitted drugs
    Dextromethorphan
    Diphenoxylate
    Beta-2 agonists (aerosol forms):
       Bitolterol
       Orciprenaline
       Rimiterol
       Salbutamol
       Terbutaline

[a] Urinary caffeine levels above 12 µg/ml are considered as doping. This level is easily reached
by 8 cups of coffee Items that containe caffeine and their urine caffeine levels are: 2 cups
coffee = 3–6 µg/ml; 2 colas = 1 1/2–3 µg/ml; 1 No-Doze = 3–6 µg/ml; 1 APC, Empirin,
Anacin = 2–3 µg/ml

Note   This table is not a complete list The USOC Drug Hotline (800-233-0373) should be
consulted for further information

Reprinted with permission of the U.S Olympic Committee, Drug Control Program, Committee on
Substance Abuse Research and Education. Copyright 1986

Chapter 2

NUTRITIONAL ERGOGENIC AIDS — MACRONUTRIENTS

I. INTRODUCTION

Nutritional ergogenic aids fall into three major categories: macronutrient manipulations, essential micronutrient and intermediate metabolite supplementation, and addition of other dietary substances. Results from studies on each type of nutrient will be examined, and if possible, guidelines on use of nutrients will be given to foster applicability of latest data.

For the purpose of this book, macronutrients are defined as water, electrolytes, carbohydrates, proteins, and fats, with daily requirements of each in the range of grams. Each of these macronutrients is of primary importance for human athletic performance. Other reviews that relate macronutrients and performance have been published.[8,30-37] Macronutrient manipulations designed to improve performance will be discussed, with emphasis on guidelines.

II. MACRONUTRIENT MANIPULATION

A. HYDRATION AND ELECTROLYTE REPLACEMENT

Skeletal muscle and blood have water contents of 80% and 93%, respectively.[38] Homeostasis of blood osmolality, body temperature, and plasma electrolyte (sodium, potassium, and chloride ions) levels is maintained to a greater degree than any other physiological parameter during exercise, along with pH.[38,39] Fluid loss during exercise, primarily from sweat, is one of the major causes of fatigue.[36,39-41] Thus, hydration of athletes is vital for performance.

Factors that argue for close attention to hydration and electrolyte repletion during exercise include

1. High ambient temperature (>30°C)
2. High relative humidity (>80%)
3. High loss rates of sweating (>2 l/h)
4. High body temperatures (>2°C from resting level)
5. Length of exercise (>1 h)
6. Untrained subjects
7. Exercise intensity (close to maximal oxygen capacity (VO_2max))
8. High body fat percentage
9. Heat-trapping clothing
10. Exercise underwater (swimming and scuba diving)
11. Diuretic drugs or diseases (such as uncontrolled diabetes)[36,38-43]

7

A wide range of sweat rates (over fourfold) is found among individuals.[44] Thus, if one seems to sweat more than others, special efforts to maintain hydration should be considered. Measurement of body weight immediately before and after exercise can yield the percentage of body weight lost. If loss of body weight exceeds 2%, then performance may suffer, and rehydration is indicated.[36] Thirst is a poor indicator of hydration needs. By the time one is thirsty during exercise, partial dehydration has already occurred.[36]

Sweat loss during exercise is associated with a concomitant loss of the electrolytes sodium, potassium, chloride, and magnesium.[36,38–42] Although sweat is hypotonic compared to plasma, excessive sweating (10 to 12 l over several hours) may lead to imbalances in normal electrolyte ratios, disturbing nervous system and muscular function, even to the point of ventricular fibrillation and death.[39,40] For these reasons, salt tablets have been recommended in the past to prevent sodium losses. Currently, indiscriminate use of salt tablets is discouraged, except for untrained persons losing over 7 lb of body weight as sweat per day.[40] Supplemental amounts of sodium chloride in these situations should reach 4 to 5 g daily until acclimatization has occurred. One level teaspoon of table salt contains 6 g.

Repletion of potassium and magnesium to prevent fatigue from electrolyte loss is also hypothesized. Various electrolyte replacement drinks have appeared to negate losses, but reports on exercise performance following ingestion of these drinks are equivocal, although some reports show some benefits.[39,40]

1. Guidelines for Hydration

The American College of Sports Medicine has published a position statement for prevention of thermal injury during distance running in the heat.[45] Ingestion of 400 to 600 ml of cold water 15 to 20 min before the event, followed by intake of 100 to 200 ml every 2 to 3 km was suggested, which gives a total intake of 1.4 to 4.2 l/h.[45] In practice, intakes greater than 2 l/h are unlikely.[36] These guidelines are appropriate for long-term exercise (>1 h) when the factors listed above are in effect.

Short-term (<30 min), intense exercise has not benefitted from rehydration.[46] Also, ingestion of large volumes of fluids during intense exercise (>80% VO_2max) usually results in nausea and vomiting.

In ultra-long-distance events or repeated exercise in the heat, consumption of water alone has led to overhydration (hyponatremia) in a few cases.[47] In these circumstances, electrolyte solutions are more appropriate. Sodium chloride is the preferred solute, at low, hypotonic concentrations of 10 to 25 mmol/l, which are present in most commercially available sports drinks. Drinks with higher sodium contents (30 to 90 mmol/l) should be avoided during exercise because their taste usually limits intake.

After exercise, electrolyte repletion should be accomplished easily by normal diets. For those who consume a low-salt diet, adding table salt to foods may be beneficial. Electrolyte replacement drinks are also adequate for consumption after an event.

Importantly, consumption of water or water/electrolyte mixtures under conditions where exercise performance has not benefited has never been shown to lead to decreases in performance.[36] Thus, even if sports drinks or water are consumed unnecessarily, performance will not be compromised.

In summary, water repletion during exercise appears to be the most important nutritional ergogenic aid yet studied,[36,38–43] and is recommended by every expert on exercise performance.

B. CARBOHYDRATE NUTRITION AND PERFORMANCE

1. Glycogen Supercompensation (Carbohydrate Loading)

It is now clear that the availability of carbohydrates to muscles is a limiting factor for prolonged, strenuous exercise.[37,48–51] Carbohydrates are presented to muscles primarily as the monosaccharide glucose, with minor contributions from glycerol and other sugars. Storage of glucose is found mainly in liver and muscles as a branched-chain polymer named glycogen. When muscle glycogen stores are depleted and blood glucose levels are significantly lowered, fatigue results.[37,51] Since carbohydrates are the major source of energy at exercise intensities of $\geq 70\%$ VO_2max and are about 50% of energy sources at lower intensities,[52] carbohydrate availability to exercising muscles is obviously of paramount importance for maintenance of performance. Thus, loss of carbohydrates ranks directly behind dehydration and loss of electrolytes as a major cause of fatigue. Carbohydrate status is directly related to dietary intake rather than other variables. Thus, nutritional modulation of carbohydrate status has been explored in some detail in order to enhance or prolong performance. Increasing duration of carbohydrate availability to exercising muscles can be accomplished by increasing glycogen storage above usual amounts, termed glycogen supercompensation, or more popularly, carbohydrate loading.

During long-term exercise lasting more than 2 h, muscle glycogen stores are mobilized first.[37,49–51,53] When muscle glycogen stores become depleted, blood glucose becomes the major source of carbohydrate for exercising muscles.[37,49–51] Liver glycogen, gluconeogenesis (formation of glucose) from amino acids, and exogenous dietary sources of carbohydrate then become the chief energy source for exercising muscle. When blood glucose levels fall below normal physiological levels (<70 mg/dl) and muscle glycogen levels are depleted, fatigue ensues.

Levels of muscle and liver glycogen are one determinant of muscular endurance.[37,50,54–59] Higher levels of tissue glycogen are associated with greater physical performance.[37,50,54,55,60–69] Two types of dietary regimens have been used to optimize glycogen stores.

a. Classical (Astrand) Regimen

First, the Astrand (or "classical") regimen achieves muscle glycogen supercompensation by a period of glycogen depletion followed by repletion, wherein an athlete combines exercise with changes in carbohydrate intake.[58,70–73] This procedure lasts approximately 1 week and is done to prepare for a single event, usually a competition. From 1 week to 2 or 3 d before the scheduled event, exhaustive exercise is coupled with a low carbohydrate diet (0 to 10% of calorie intake) to deplete glycogen stores. Next, a high carbohydrate/low fat diet (80 to 90% of caloric intake from carbohydrates) is consumed, with little or no exercise until the event. This type of regimen has been shown to supersaturate tissue glycogen levels, leading to increased long-term aerobic performance.[58,70] However, the Astrand regimen is stressful to many individuals, especially diabetics, and may cause disturbances in glucose metabolism or ECG readings.[54] Dietary manipulations are not simple, and to achieve desired intakes, considerable dietary expertise is necessary.

b. Sherman/Costill Method

The second method of carbohydrate loading (Sherman/Costill method) is currently the preferred method, and consists of keeping the body saturated with carbohydrates in order to maximize tissue glycogen levels. To accomplish this goal, an athlete must usually consume 60 to 70% of dietary calories as carbohydrates (up to 600 g of carbohydrates daily). This amount of carbohydrate-rich food is equivalent to about 2 loaves of bread, or 3 cups of sugar, or 15 baked potatoes, or 12 cups of rice daily. To train for a particular event, exercise is tapered starting a week before the event. Every second day, the amount of exercise is halved until no exercise is performed the day before the event. The high carbohydrate diet is consumed throughout this period. Research has shown that this second method of glycogen supercompensation yields tissue glycogen levels equivalent to the Astrand regimen, and performance is also improved to the same extent.[37,49–51,53–55,74–77] The potential drawbacks of the depletion phase of the Astrand regime are not encountered with this second method. Training for repetitive events and dietary manipulations are simpler, meaning greater practical success. Table 1 lists sports events for which carbohydrate loading is or is not indicated.

c. Carbohydrate Loading — Indications

Carbohydrate loading is indicated for events lasting 1.5 to 2 h or longer.[37,49,50] Benefits of carbohydrate loading for shorter events or more anaerobic exercises (like weightlifting) are unclear at this time.[65,78,79] In addition, a diet high in carbohydrates may help prevent overtraining.[37,80,81] An increasing number of athletes are consuming more carbohydrates and fewer fats in their daily diets, as exhibited by the recent emphasis on carbohydrate nutrition seen in popular fitness magazines.

Carbohydrate loading can easily be accomplished inexpensively with foods alone, providing that an athlete has at least basic nutritional knowledge. The availability of purified carbohydrates has produced a plethora of commercial products designed for use in carbohydrate loading or in supplying carbohydrates for exercise endurance. Such products offer convenient preparation, less fecal and intestinal residue, and no fat or protein calories, but they are more costly than food sources containing equal amounts of carbohydrate. Products

TABLE 1
Sports Activities Suitable for Glycogen Supercompensation
(Carbohydrate Loading)

More suitable events	Less suitable events
Marathon	Football games
Triathlon	Basketball games
Cross-country skiing	Baseball games
Ultra-endurance events	Runs <10 km
Soccer	Downhill ski runs
Cycling time trials	Walking and hiking
Rock climbing	Most swimming events
Mountain climbing	Weight lifting
Long distance swimming	Most track and field events
Long distance canoe or kayak events	Sprinting
Endurance events lasting more than	Most rowing events
90 min with sustained 70 to 90%	
VO$_2$max	
Practice sessions lasting >2 hr	
involving constant activity	
Short-term exhaustive exercise after	
prolonged endurance events	

containing maltodextrin or glucose polymers have been reported to be slightly more effective than foods such as pasta for supplying muscle glycogen storage and improving performance.[54,82,83] Starches (complex carbohydrates) are preferred for glycogen replenishment prior to exercise, although simple sugars also can increase glycogen stores.[84] For greater details on glycogen supercompensation, the reader is referred to other reviews.[31,37,48–50,53–55,69,80]

2. High-Carbohydrate Pre-Exercise Meal

In addition to glycogen supercompensation, a pre-exercise meal (3 to 4 h before an event) containing ≥300 g carbohydrates has been shown to further enhance exercise performance by 15%.[37,50,77,85–89] Smaller amounts of carbohydrates in pre-exercise meals did not improve exercise performance.[88] The pre-exercise meal should consist mostly of low-fiber, complex carbohydrates (starches) instead of simple sugars to minimize adverse metabolic changes in carbohydrate metabolism.

3. Carbohydrate Replenishment During Exercise

As stated previously, availability of glucose to exercising muscles is a major factor delaying fatigue in long-term exercise. A high-carbohydrate diet, glycogen supercompensation, and a high-carbohydrate pre-exercise meal can all benefit long-term exercise performance. Perhaps an equally or even more effective way to maintain performance is supplementation with exogenous dietary carbohydrates *during* exercise.[37,48–51]

Numerous studies have examined carbohydrate feeding during exercise performance.[37,48–51,54,69,82,83,90–117] Most have found increased time before fatigue, increased work output, and improved performance after prolonged exercise. The magnitude of benefits varies depending on type of exercise, duration, intensity, training status of individuals, previous dietary intake, type of carbohydrate ingested, osmolality of ingested carbohydrate, dosage schedule, and other factors. However, research shows a clear consensus that onset of fatigue can be delayed significantly, ranging from extending exercise time a few minutes to being able to achieve an otherwise unattainable finish.

For well-fed, well-trained, elite individuals, carbohydrate repletion during exercise lasting 3 h or more is beneficial.[51] Benefits for shorter events can be seen when carbohydrate status is not optimum. Amateur athletes show improvements in events lasting ≥2 h, while untrained individuals show benefits in events lasting ≥1.5 h.[51]

Carbohydrate replenishment during exercise is most easily achieved according to the guidelines by consuming commercially available sports drinks. Almost all products have been designed to supply water, carbohydrates, and electrolytes in sufficient quantities to provide practical, useful repletion. It is important to choose a drink that is palatable, to encourage consumption. Carbohydrate-containing drinks may be used before, during, and after exercise[37,51,53] or may be consumed just before onset of fatigue (after 1 to 2 h of endurance exercise), with benefits still likely.[37,51,115] About 1 to 1.5 cups (8 to 12 fl oz or 250 ml) of sports drink should be consumed every 15 to 20 min. A total of 40 to 70 g carbohydrates per hour should be consumed to supply sufficient glucose to maintain performance between 70 to 90% VO_2max.[51]

Another alternative to sports drinks is to dilute any fruit juice 1:1 with water, and add a teaspoon of salt per liter (quart). This will closely approximate carbohydrate, electrolyte, and osmolality values of commercially available sports drinks.

4. Post-Exercise Carbohydrate Replenishment

Glycogen resynthesis following strenuous exercise that depletes glycogen stores can determine how soon an athlete may resume optimal performance.[37,53] This scenario is important for hastened recovery, particularly during multi-day athletic events, when optimal performance must be maintained. Studies have found that a diet rich in carbohydrates (>300 g/24 h) can replete muscle glycogen stores to normal or supercompensated levels in 20 to 24 h.[37,53,84,118] To accomplish this task, the following conditions should be satisfied:

1. Initiate carbohydrate feeding immediately (<2 h) after cessation of exercise;[37,53,119]
2. Consume about 50 g carbohydrates (equivalent to 0.7 g glucose/kg body weight) every 2 h for the first 4 to 6 h post-exercise, and 500 to 700 g total carbohydrates in 20 to 24 h following exercise;[37,53,84,120–123]
3. Consume simple carbohydrates (sugars like glucose or sucrose or high glycemic index foods) rather than complex carbohydrates (low glycemic index foods or fructose) during the first 6 h post-exercise;[37,53,84,122–126]

4. In events causing complete exhaustion, eccentric exercise or muscle soreness/damage, consume even more carbohydrates for optimal glycogen repletion.[37,53,127-129]

Benefits from rapid and full replenishment of glycogen levels by post-exercise dietary carbohydrate intake include faster recuperation, faster return to training, and maintenance of exercise performance (prevention of impaired performance) in strenuous daily events (such as Tour de France cycling races).

5. Other Forms of Carbohydrate Supplementation

Fructose 1,6-diphosphate (FDP), an intermediate metabolite of glycolysis, has been used to restore glycolytic energy production in extreme conditions of muscular and cardiac performance (acidosis, ischemia, hypoxia, peripheral vascular disease, exertional claudication).[130] Exogenously administering FDP can restore FDP levels decreased by a pH-dependent inhibition of phosphofructokinase (PFK) by direct feedback stimulation of PFK activity and by entering the glycolytic pathway.[131] Infusions of FDP to animals in cardiac arrest or severe shock (conditions of extreme acidosis and muscular ischemia) have produced improvements in cardiovascular functions and survival.[130] However, compared to a placebo period, infusion of 200 mg/kg FDP into 10 males with peripheral vascular disease and stable exertional claudication did not affect heart rate, blood pressure, gas exchange measurements, time to onset of claudication, peak levels of lactate and 2,3-diphosphoglycerate, or exercise capacity.[130] Thus, infusion of FDP may not be useful in conditions where extreme, life-threatening hypoxia or ischemia are not present.

6. Carbohydrates as Ergogenic Aids — Summary

Maintenance of glucose supply to exercising muscle is essential for optimal performance in long-term, strenuous exercise. Glucose supply may be prolonged and enhanced by four types of dietary manipulations involving carbohydrate intake, as shown in Table 2.

Carbohydrate-rich diets are helpful before and after exercise. During exercise, intake of commercially available sports drinks repletes water, electrolytes, and carbohydrates with a single foodstuff. Thus, three major causes of fatigue can be counteracted simultaneously.[48] In conclusion, available research has demonstrated ergogenic benefits from ingestion of sports drinks containing carbohydrate and electrolytes for strenuous endurance exercises. Effects on other events and exercises are less clear.

C. PROTEIN INTAKE AND PHYSICAL PERFORMANCE

Athletes, especially weightlifters, have imbedded in their psyche a desire to consume large amounts of protein. This desire stems from the tradition, fostered by centuries of anecdotal, but not totally correct, conclusions that meat ingestion increases muscle mass. Central questions concerning dietary protein and ergogenesis include (1) whether supplemental or high protein intake provides additional energy for exercise performance, and (2) whether supple-

TABLE 2
Dietary Manipulations of Carbohydrate Intake Known to Prolong or Enhance Long-term Exercise Performance

1. Carbohydrate loading (glycogen supercompensation)
2. Pre-exercise, carbohydrate-rich meal
3. Carbohydrate ingestion during exercise (sports drinks)
4. Post-exercise replenishment of glycogen

mental or high protein intake enhances accretion of muscle mass in weightlifters and strength athletes, and thereby improve strength and power.

1. Protein and Energy

It is now apparent that protein catabolism can account for 5 to 10% of energy production during endurance exercise.[35,132,133] Thus, proteins (and amino acids) are a minor source of energy for exercising muscles. At this time, there is insufficient research to determine whether high protein intakes will benefit endurance performance. However, various studies on protein metabolism of long-distance endurance runners suggest that protein needs are elevated 50 to 100% over the USRDA of 0.8 g protein/kg/d.[35,134] This need translates into approximately 1.5 g protein/kg/d (105 g protein daily for a 70-kg person) during the first month after initiation or increase of exercise workload. Thereafter, and for well-trained endurance athletes, 1.2 to 1.4 g protein/kg/d (84 to 98 g protein/d) is sufficient to provide a positive nitrogen (protein) metabolism.[35,134]

In summary, there is no convincing evidence that increased dietary protein intake provides a significant ergogenic effect for long-term endurance exercise. However, increased protein intake may be necessary during short-term increases of workload to prevent negative alterations in nitrogen metabolism.

2. Protein Intake and Muscle Mass

Attainment of muscular hypertrophy is one form of ergogenesis, in the sense that increased muscular size can eventually confer greater strength, and thus, enhanced performance in weightlifting, bodybuilding, strength events, and certain sports (especially football). Currently, many athletes and nonathletes are seeking to increase muscle mass and/or strength, and dietary manipulations that can accelerate muscular hypertrophy are in high demand. Hypothetically, enough data has been accumulated that general conclusions have been offered about the amount of dietary protein needed for muscle hypertrophy.[135] One pound of muscle contains about 100 g of protein.[135] For a theoretical increase in muscle mass of 1 lb/week, at least 14 g of additional protein per day are required (100 ÷ 7 = 14), along with additional calories.[135] This increase in protein and calories can be met by increasing food consumption, since 4000 kcal daily with 20% of calories derived from protein supplies approximately 2.8 g protein/kg/d, or 200 g. This level is consistent with research showing muscle mass increases during training.[35,135,136]

Studies on strength or muscular development after increased protein intake are few and contradictory. Protein supplements or high intake of meats without exercise have been shown not to increase muscle mass in a specific manner.[137] The early works of Kraut studied protein intakes of 55 g, and later, 100 g protein daily on two undernourished subjects undergoing vigorous muscular training.[138] A subsequent study of two subjects lifting weights reported a doubling of strength in three months with a protein intake of 2.0 g/kg/d.[139] These subjects were then fed a diet with less protein, and no further gains were noted.[139] Kraut et al. concluded that protein supplementation aided increased muscle mass and strength induced by heavy training. Two double-blind studies indicated that supplemental protein increased the strength of college athletes in training, but no experimental details or references were listed.[140]

On the other hand, studies with acceptable controls have not found significant differences in strength and power between control and protein-supplemented (25 g/d or 0.69 g/kg/d) groups.[141,142] One possible drawback to these findings was the short experimental periods for these studies (less than 6 weeks) or the low dose of protein supplemented.

Other studies have found alterations in protein metabolism for high protein intakes that may offer benefits for muscular hypertrophy. When three sedentary subjects received a high-protein diet (372% RDA) for 2 months, nitrogen balance remained significantly positive throughout the study period.[143] A report by Consolazio et al. found large increases in nitrogen retention (32 vs. 7 g) and lean body mass (3.3 vs. 1.2 kg) after a 40-d period of exercise in two groups of subjects given 2.8 or 1.4 g protein/kg/d (350 vs. 175% RDA).[136] Likewise, Marable reported that a diet providing 300% RDA of protein compared to 100% RDA improved nitrogen retention (104 vs. 70 mg/kg).[144] Dragan et al. noted increases in strength (5%) and lean body mass (6%) in weightlifters after protein intake was increased from 2.2 to 3.5 g/kg/d (275 to 435% RDA).[145] A nutritionally complete liquid supplement containing protein and supplying 500 kcal/d was given to a group of 15 competitive weightlifters at the Swedish Sports Medicine Center in Englewood, Colorado.[146] Fifteen unsupplemented competitive weightlifters served as a control group. Both groups consumed a self-selected diet and did not use anabolic steroids. After 15 weeks, the supplemented group gained significantly greater body weight (7.1 vs. 3.5 lb) and lost significantly more body fat (−0.91 vs. −0.30%) than the control group. Finally, in older men initiating a resistance exercise program, Frontera et al. measured increases in thigh muscle sizes and urine creatine excretion (a crude measure of muscle mass), but found no changes in thigh muscle strength after a dietary protein supplement of 0.33 g/kg/d was supplied.[147]

Taken together, these results suggest that higher dietary protein intakes (≥300% RDA, or ≥2.4 g protein/kg/d, or ≥168 g protein/d) may facilitate muscular hypertrophy. These results tend to corroborate widespread anecdotal beliefs of weightlifters that high dietary protein intakes are essential for maximum muscular development during resistance training.

Obviously, these results do not yet prove that high protein intakes improve muscle mass formation during resistance training, but suggest that further research differentiate whether observed results are due to the caloric value of additional protein or more specific effects. Certainly, high protein diets do not impede muscular hypertrophy in resistance training.

3. Dietary Protein Supplements — Sophisticated Variety of Choices

The use of protein supplements by athletes for strength training has become entrenched and is continually fostered. Proponents of protein supplements claim the advantages listed in Table 3. These claimed advantages seem to outweigh the disadvantage of higher cost of protein supplements compared to foodstuffs for consumers.

Upon closer examination, protein powders are a more cost-effective source of protein per dollar than vegetables, grains, nuts, cheeses, fish, and most beef foodstuffs. Protein powders are less cost-effective than powdered milk, milk, eggs, chicken, or pork. Except for nonfat powdered milk, the foods that are less costly than protein powders contain considerable quantities of fat, which contribute to undesirable intake of excess calories for certain athletes wishing to reduce body fat levels (such as bodybuilders). Powdered milk contains much lactose, which may cause disturbances in lactose-intolerant individuals. In addition, for the cost of one or two restaurant dinners or a 1 week supply of meat ($20.00), an individual can consume 50 g/d of supplemental protein for at least an entire month from protein powder. Thus, athletes view protein powders as a cost effective and convenient source of additional dietary protein. For these reasons, demand for such products, regardless of justification, will remain.

Lately, two other forms of protein supplementation have appeared. Protein hydrolysates and free-form amino acid mixtures have captured a large segment of the protein supplement market. Protein hydrolysates offer a predigested form of protein(s), and have been used clinically for enteral feeding of hospitalized patients.[148] Enzymic hydrolysis of source proteins is normally utilized, avoiding the losses of serine, threonine, tryptophan, and cysteine as well as salt content found with acid hydrolysis. As a result, an ever-increasing number of hydrolysates are commercially available. Some companies claim improved or hastened absorption over dietary proteins or even amino acid mixtures for their products, although no evidence using commercial dietary supplement products has been reported. Clever advertising literature and numerous testimonials support marketing of these products. Costs of protein hydrolysate products range from two to five times the cost of protein powders for equivalent amounts of nitrogenous material. However, no reports of improved performance or weight gain due to protein hydrolysate use on athletes can be found in peer-reviewed literature.

Amino acid mixtures have come into vogue within the last 10 years because of the availability of bulk amounts of food-grade L-amino acids. Most purified amino acids (commonly referred to as free-form) are produced by large-scale

TABLE 3
Purported Advantages of Purified Protein Supplements Compared to Whole Foods

1 Ensure adequate protein intake if diet is inadequate
2 Replace fat-laden dietary protein sources
3 Convenient preparation and storage of protein source
4 Long shelf-life and stability
5 Additional source of energy
6 Addition of other nutrients to enhance food value of supplement (for some products)
7 Comparable or lower cost than many high-protein foods

microbial fermentation processes in Japan, accounting for the great expense of free-form amino acids as a sole dietary nitrogen source. Mixtures of amino acids (as pharmaceutical grade) have been used clinically for intravenous and enteral feeding of hospitalized patients since the 1950s.[148-151] In addition, long-term (6 month) oral feedings of free-form amino acids as the sole source of nitrogen in a chemically defined diet to normal healthy males have illustrated the safety of this form of protein nutriture and the ability of the subjects to thrive.[152] Proponents of free-form amino acid mixtures claim that absorption is complete with no fecal residue, absorption of nitrogen is more rapid than from proteins, amino acid compositions can be manipulated to optimize energy or protein synthesis for users, and various physiological parameters can be influenced (e.g., hormone release). All these claims arise from use of indirectly supportive references taken from peer-reviewed literature. However, objective testing of commercial formulas available to athletes regarding effects on physical performance has not been reported.

One recent report by Lowry et al.[153] described urinary excretion of nitrogen, 3-methylhistidine, and creatine before and after submaximal (40% of maximal) bicycle exercise. Subjects deriving nutrition solely from intravenous feeding of crystalline free-form amino acids and glucose exhibited lower levels of nitrogen loss and 3-methylhistidine loss than during a period of oral feeding. These results indicated that infused free-form amino acids and glucose provided sufficient substrates to spare myofibrillar proteins during exercise. Thus, exogenous free-form amino acids have been demonstrated to possess the ability to prevent exercise-induced protein catabolism. The applicability of these findings to oral use of free-form amino acid supplements remains to be determined. Otherwise, no direct objective data exists to support or contradict the claims of proponents of free-form amino acid supplements. Research into the effects of free-form amino acid mixtures is needed, if only to confront the increasing use of these supplements. Effects of differing compositions of mixtures present another large variable for researchers.

4. Summary of Ergogenic Effects of Protein
Compared to the study of carbohydrates and endurance performance, the study of protein nutrition and muscular hypertrophy/strength is grossly inad-

equate to yield definite conclusions or guidelines. The basic question of whether increased dietary protein improves nitrogen metabolism by a simple caloric effect or by more specific effects unique to amino acids remains to be explored. However, a consensus is emerging that initiation of increased exercise workloads (endurance or strength training) probably increases protein requirements, at least for a relatively short time period of 1 to 2 months. Whether improvements in nitrogen metabolism from high dietary protein intakes will be prolonged is not yet clear. Also, interaction of protein with total caloric intake suggests that higher caloric intakes may spare the need for high intakes of protein.[35,134,146,154] Furthermore, a diet high in complex carbohydrates combined with a protein supplement enriched in amino acids involved in gluconeogenesis (e.g., alanine) has been suggested to help maintain muscular ATP production.[133]

At this time, there is almost no evidence to indicate that high-protein diets are unsafe for normal adults.[35,135,155] There is certainly no evidence that strength athletes who consume high protein diets (and who do not use anabolic steroids) have increased incidence of hepatic or renal dysfunctions.[35] Although excess dietary protein is not recommended for patients with liver or kidney failure,[155] these situations do not apply to the average weight lifter. Studies in which animals were fed a very high protein intake (80% of calories) for over half their lifespans noted only minor negative effects (enlargement of liver mitochondria).[156] Thus, high protein diets *per se* are generally safe.

At present, it is prudent and defensible to ensure a dietary protein intake of about 100 g/d for a 70-kg endurance athlete after an increase in workload for at least one month. Strength athletes (weightlifters) may likewise ensure a dietary protein intake of 112 to 178 g/d for 70-kg individuals during the first 6 to 8 weeks after an increase in workload.

D. FATS AND ERGOGENESIS

Fats (as plasma free fatty acids) represent the major source for muscular energy at low intensities, and training enhances the ability to metabolize fats for muscular energy during exercise.[52,157] While fats are well known as major energy sources for muscles, the role of dietary fat in ergogenesis has been almost completely ignored because even persons with very low body fat store huge amounts of energy as triglycerides in intramuscular and adipose tissue deposits.[52,157] Thus, high intakes of dietary fat (60 to 80% of caloric intake) have experienced almost no beneficial effects on muscular exercise performance and may actually decrease performance relative to high-carbohydrate diets.[52,157]

However, recent evidence has suggested that two types of dietary fat possess interesting properties that may benefit exercise performance if manipulated correctly. These fats are omega-3 fatty acids and medium-chain triglycerides (MCTs).

1. Omega-3 Fatty Acids — Performance Implications

Omega-3 fatty acids are long chain, polyunsaturated fatty acids with a double bond on the third carbon from the end of the molecule. Omega-3 fatty acids manifest biological functions via conversion to eicosanoids (prostaglandin, thromboxanes, and leukotrienes) that have profound physiological effects.[158-160] In addition, omega-3 fatty acids compete with the omega-6 fatty acid, arachidonic acid, which forms a series of pro-inflammatory, pro-aggregatory eicosanoids (so-called "bad" prostaglandins).[158] Biological effects of omega-3 fatty acids range from increased bleeding times, decreased platelet adhesiveness, reduced plasma triglyceride and cholesterol levels, improved membrane fluidity (especially in erythrocytes), and changes in vascular endothelial eicosanoids to more antiinflammatory compounds.[158-160] Furthermore, omega-3 fatty acids promote formation of prostaglandin E_1, which stimulates and makes possible somatotropin release.[161-165] Potential mechanisms whereby omega-3 fatty acids can influence exercise performance thus are not mediated by their calorie value, but rather, by formation of regulatory hormones governing basic physiological components related to exercise. Table 4 lists some postulated mechanisms of ergogenic effects of omega-3 fatty acids.

In healthy humans made ischemic with a thigh tourniquet, infusion of prostaglandin E1 (PGE_1) (produced by omega-3 fatty acids) produced a blood flow 2.5 times greater than placebo infusions.[166] In addition, blood ratio of lactate/pyruvate more closely resembled normal ratios after PGE_1 infusions. Patients with occlusive arterial disease (intermittent claudication) exhibited increased maximum walking distance and pain free walking distance after PGE_1 injections compared to placebo injections.[167] PGE_1 infusion in a diabetic patient scheduled for leg amputation improved vasodilation of the leg artery so that amputation was unnecessary.[168] PGE_1, produced from gamma linolenic (GLA) and dihomo-gamma linolenic acid (DGLA, an omega-3 fatty acid),[169,170] has repeatedly exhibited potent anti-platelet aggregatory and vasodilatory properties. Vasodilatory properties are of interest to athletes to improve flow of oxygen and nutrients to muscle tissues during exercise. GLA supplements have been widely available for many years, but until recently have not been applied to exercise performance.

a. Human Studies

Studies on human athletes have utilized Eicomax®, a commercially available blend of fish oils and vegetable oils supplying GLA, eicosapentaenoic acid (EPA), and docosahexaenoic acid (DHA) (omega-3 fatty acids).[171] In 1988, the entire football team of Liberty University was tested for both cardiovascular and strength parameters before and after an 8-week period during the football season (peak fitness conditions). After supplementation with 8 capsules of Eicomax® daily, bench press repetitions increased 10.2%, number of chin-ups increased 9.3%, vertical jumps increased 2.6%, 300-yd shuttle times decreased 3.0%, and heart rate one min after the shuttle run decreased 8.6%.[171] These results in an open-field trial suggested omega-3 fatty acid supplementation was associated with improvements in both strength and aerobic performance. A double-blind, placebo-controlled study of the Boise State football team during off-season conditioning employed Eicomax® or olive oil placebos. After 8 weeks a significant increase in bench press 1-repetition maximum (strength)

TABLE 4
Postulated Mechanisms of Ergogenic Effects from Omega-3 Fatty Acids

1. Improved delivery of oxygen and nutrients to muscles and other tissues from ↓ blood viscosity, capillary vasodilation, and ↑ erythrocyte deformability yielding greater tissue perfusion
2. Enhanced aerobic metabolism (↑ VO_2max) from improved delivery of O_2
3. Enhanced release of somatotropin in response to normal stimuli (exercise, sleep, hunger) may have anabolic/recovery effects
4. Reduction of inflammation caused by muscular fatigue and overexertion (allows recovery to proceed sooner than normal)
5. Modulation of eicosanoid synthesis to favor anti-inflammatory and rheological properties

was observed (+6 vs. +1%).[171] Other anecdotal cases and use by professional football teams appeared to associate Eicomax® with simultaneous improvements in both strength and cardiovascular performance.[171] These results led to endorsement of Eicomax® by the NFL Players Association (NFLPA) as a realistic nutritional alternative to anabolic steroids.[171]

Finally, a study from Western Washington University divided 32 healthy young males into four groups.[172] One group served as controls, another was supplemented with menhaden fish oil plus salmon steaks for a daily omega-3 fatty acid intake of 4 g/d (equivalent to 12 capsules/d of fish oil supplements), another group participated in an aerobic exercise program, and the last group participated in the exercise program and ingested omega-3 supplements. After 10 weeks, VO_2max improved slightly in the control group (+4.5%), more so in the omega-3 fatty acid supplement group (+11%), and significantly in both exercise groups (+23 and +20%). Ventilation anaerobic threshold (VAT as percent VO_2max) showed a slight decrease in the control group, and significant increases in the other groups. Fish oil (omega-3 fatty acid) supplementation was associated with slight improvements in aerobic metabolism, although quantitative benefits were greater from aerobic exercise. This study illustrated that postulated mechanisms of omega-3 fatty acid supplementation mimic effects of aerobic exercise in both theory and practice.

In summary, dietary modulation of omega-3 fatty acid intake shows promise to manipulate regulatory hormones, and producing ergogenic benefits for both aerobic and strength performance. Effects mimic benefits of aerobic exercise, supporting the postulated mechanism of action.

2. Medium-Chain Triglycerides (MCTs) — Ergogenic Properties

Another class of dietary lipids holds promise as an ergogenic aid. Medium-chain triglycerides (MCTs) are found in human milk, coconut oil, and palm kernel oil and consist of saturated fatty acids with chain lengths of 6, 8, 10, and 12 carbons.[173–175] Unlike other fats, MCTs possess unique physiological properties that strongly indicate a need for further study as an ergogenic aid.

MCTs are rapidly absorbed, and enter portal blood (not the lymphatic system), where they are readily taken up by the liver.[173,174] MCTs are rapidly oxidized to produce ketone bodies and cellular energy,[174,176] and do not rely upon carnitine to enter mitochondria.[174] Metabolism of MCTs resembles the effects of carbohydrate oxidation rather than fat oxidation.[174] MCTs seem to mobilize body fat stores[177-179] and increase resting metabolic rate.[176,180,181] Furthermore, MCTs are not easily stored as body fat,[177,178,182] and spare lean muscle mass.[183] Both MCTs and coconut oil (48% MCTs) are nonatherogenic.[184]

Thus, MCTs have been shown to possess at least four properties of vital interest to exercise performance: (1) they are a readily available energy source; (2) mobilize body fat stores; (3) increase metabolic rate; and (4) spare lean muscle mass. These properties are desirable for both long-term endurance athletes as well as strength athletes. MCTs have been in human clinical use for over 30 years with excellent safety as components of enteral feeding supplements.[175] Commercial availability is rapidly increasing, with MCT oil supplements available in most health food stores. Being completely saturated, MCT oils are the most stable edible oils known. At this time, proper dosages are not clear, but these will probably range from 2 to 4 tablespoons daily.

Potential applications of MCTs include their use as pre-exercise meals to improve endurance performance, to prevent muscle mass loss from strenuous exercise of any type (especially ultra-endurance events and weight lifting), to recover from immobilizing injuries with less loss of muscle mass, and to aid in body fat loss without lean body mass loss. Thus, replacement of part of dietary lipid intake with MCT oil holds great promise as a safe and effective ergogenic aid.

Chapter 3

MICRONUTRIENT SUPPLEMENTATION AND ERGOGENESIS — VITAMINS

I. INTRODUCTION

Micronutrients include dietary compounds that are normally found in or required by the body in minor quantities. Dietary doses usually range from nanogram (ng) to milligram (mg) ranges of intake. Essential vitamins, minerals, and metabolic intermediates are the most common micronutrients. This chapter will explore effects of micronutrients on exercise and sports performance.

II. WATER-SOLUBLE VITAMINS

A. B VITAMINS

B vitamins are a class of structurally different compounds utilized as enzyme cofactors in human intermediary metabolism. Table 1 lists physiological functions of B vitamins that relate to exercise performance. During the 1920s to 1940s, reports of effects of B-vitamin supplementation on human performance appeared. B vitamins had recently been discovered, and World War II also prompted funding of such studies. Some initial results of B-complex or individual B-vitamin supplementation showed increases in performance.[185-196] These studies all suffered from lack of control, lack of statistical analysis, or crude measurements of performance, and thus are not conclusive evidence that B-vitamin supplementation aids performance in nondeficient individuals.[197-200] Other reports during this period did not reveal significant effects from B-vitamin supplementation.[195,199-205] These studies, although adequately controlled, used doses that were not higher than normal daily intakes or only two to three times that of present RDAs.[195,200-205] They also suffered from crude measurements of performance. However, a consensus that B-vitamin supplementation was not necessary or productive was reached, creating little incentive for initiating more extensive studies.

1. Thiamine (Vitamin B₁)

Vitamin B_1 (thiamine) supplementation (900 mg/d) for 3 d to 15 trained cyclists led to consistent and significant increases in anaerobic thresholds (lower blood lactate and glucose levels, lower heart rates) during maximal cycle ergometry.[206]

2. Riboflavin (Vitamin B₂)

Acute vitamin B_2 (riboflavin) supplementation (10 mg/d) to athletes led to a "...moderate lowering of neuromuscular irritability (musculi vastus

TABLE 1
Functions of B Vitamins Related to Exercise

Vitamin B₁ (Thiamine)

Role: energy production from foodstuffs, especially carbohydrates

Function: coenzyme for transketolase (pentose phosphate pathway); pyruvate dehydrogenase and α-ketoglutarate dehydrogenases (entry of acetyl groups and α-ketoglutarate into tricarboxylic acid cycle)

Needs: 0 5 mg per 1000 kcalories

Deficiency Symptoms:

(early): fatigue, loss of appetite, nausea, constipation, irritability, mental depression, peripheral neuropathy

(moderate, Wernicke-Korsakoff syndrome):

ataxia, loss of fine motor control, mental confusion, loss of eye coordination

(severe, beriberi): muscular weakness and atrophy, edema, heart failure.

Vitamin B₂ (Riboflavin)

Role: energy production and cellular respiration

Function: as coenzymes flavin adenine dinucleotide (FAD) and flavin mononucleotide (FMN), vital for large number of redox reactions, releasing energy from carbohydrates, fats and proteins

Needs: 0.6 mg per 1000 kcalories

Deficiency Symptoms:

scaly dermatitis, glossitis, angular cheilitis (fissures at corners of mouth)

Niacin, Niacinamide (Nicotinic Acid, Nicotinamide, Vitamin B₃)

Roles: energy production, cellular respiration, fat synthesis

Function: as coenzymes nicotinamide adenine dinucleotide (NAD) and nicotinamide adenine dinucleotide phosphate (NADP), vital for many redox reactions, releasing energy from breakdown of carbohydrates, fats and proteins; glycogen synthesis

Needs: 6 6 Niacin Equivalents per 1000 kcalories (1 Niacin Equivalent = 1 mg niacin)

Deficiency Symptoms:

(early): muscular weakness, anorexia, indigestion, skin eruptions

(severe, pellagra): glossitis, tremors, diarrhea, dementia, dermatitis (3 D's)

Vitamin B₆ (Pyridoxine, Pyridoxal, Pyridoxamine)

Roles: amino acid metabolism and energy production

Function: as coenzyme pyridoxal phosphate (PLP), vital for numerous reactions involving transamination (transfer of amino groups), deamination (removal of amino groups), desulfuration (transfer of sulfhydryl groups), decarboxlyation (removal of organic acid group), heme formation, conversion of tryptophan to niacin, glycogen breakdown, eicosanoid synthesis

Needs: 2.0–2 2 mg per day

Deficiency Symptoms:

(early): irritability, nervousness, depression, peripheral neuropathy, sideroblastic anemia (microcytic anemia with normal or high serum iron)

(severe): peripheral neuritis, convulsions, nausea, vomiting, dermatitis, mucous membrane lesions

TABLE 1 (Continued)
Functions of B Vitamins Related to Exercise

Vitamin B_{12} (Cobalamins)

Roles:	prevention of anemia, sustains growth of rapidly dividing tissues
Function:	vital for transfer of methyl groups and folate metabolism, breakdown of odd-chain fatty acids and branched-chain amino acids
Needs:	3 0 µg per day

Deficiency Symptoms:

pernicious anemia (macrocytic anemia), with fatigue, shortness of breath, weakness; peripheral neuropathy followed by irreversible neurological damage; strict vegetarians at risk for deficiency

Folic Acid (Folacin, Folinic Acid, Pteroylglutamates)

Roles:	formation of blood cells and rapidly growing cells
Function:	primary carrier of one-carbon units used for myriad biosynthetic reactions
Needs:	0 4 mg per day

Deficiency Symptoms:

macrocytic anemia (fatigue, weakness), gastrointestinal symptoms, glossitis

Pantothenic Acid (Vitamin B_5)

Roles:	energy production from carbohydrates, fats and proteins
Function:	as coenzyme A, vital for entry of carbohydrates, fats and proteins into tricarboxylic acid cycle; and for many biosynthetic pathways
Needs:	4–7 mg per day (estimate)

Deficiency Symptoms:

deficiencies of pantothenate are generally believed to be rare; thus, if symptoms present, would mimic those for other B vitamins

Biotin (Vitamin H)

Roles:	energy production and fat metabolism
Function:	biosynthesis of fatty acids, replenishment of tricarboxylic acid cycle, gluconeogenesis
Needs:	100–300 µg per day

Deficiency Symptoms:

muscle pain, dermatitis (especially nose and mouth), depression, hair loss; large consumption of raw egg whites (>20 per day) may induce biotin deficiency

From Brown, M L , Ed., *Present Knowledge in Nutrition*, International Life Sciences Institute - Nutrition Foundation, Washington, 1990. With permission
From Devlin, T M , Ed , *Textbook of Biochemistry*, 3rd ed., Wiley-Liss, New York, 1992, 1115. With permission
From Krause, M. V and Mahan, L K , Eds , *Food, Nutrition, and Diet Therapy*, 7th ed., W B Saunders, Philadelphia, 1984, 99 With permission
From Machlin, L J , Ed., *Handbook of Vitamins*, 2nd ed Marcel Dekker, New York, 1991 With permission
From Williams, M H , *Nutritional Aspects of Human Physical Performance*, 2nd ed , Charles C Thomas, Springfield, IL, 1985, 147 With permission.

medialis and lateralis quadricipitis)..." after electrical stimulation, suggesting that improvement of muscular hyperexcitability (seen in trained athletes) may be possible, with resulting improvement of glycolytic capability and, theoretically, performance.[207]

3. Niacin (Niacinamide, Nicotinic Acid, Vitamin B₃)

Niacin (nicotinic acid or niacinamide) was found to prevent the rise in plasma-free fatty acid (FFA) levels seen during exercise.[208-210] Performance was not changed after niacin administration in those studies plus one other,[208-211] and subjects administered niacin reported greater fatigue.[211] Administration of niacin to glycogen-depleted subjects resulted in decreased endurance when compared to glycogen-depleted nonsupplemented subjects, supporting the hypothesis that FFA are an energy source during exercise and casting doubt about the use of excessive amounts of niacin alone as an ergogenic aid.[212]

4. Pyridoxine (Vitamin B₆)

Vitamin B₆ (pyridoxine) supplementation did not affect endurance of trained swimmers,[213] exercise work load after a carbohydrate-rich diet,[199] or VO₂max and peak lactate levels after supramaximal treadmill runs.[214] Pyridoxine may augment the increase in serum growth hormone induced by exercise,[215] a finding of potential importance to athletes ingesting multivitamin preparations. Supplementation of 8 mg/d of vitamin B₆ to four trained subjects undergoing carbohydrate loading manipulations caused a more rapid emptying of muscle glycogen stores during graded cycle ergometry.[216] Similar experiments on trained and untrained women consuming diets high or low in carbohydrates and supplying either 2.4 (basal) or 10.4 (supplemented) mg of pyridoxine found a similar increase in utilization of stores of glycogen and decreases in resting and exercise levels of serum FFA.[217] These two studies offer evidence for support of the hypothesis that supplemental B6 may lead to more rapid utilization of glycogen stores and less utilization of FFA during short-term submaximal exercise. If these results could be extrapolated to long-term endurance events, the findings from previous studies of no ergogenic effects after B6 supplementation may be explained.[199,213,214] Conversely, short-term anaerobic exercise that relies chiefly on glycolysis for energy (such as weightlifting), may show improvements after B6 supplementation.

5. Cobalamins (Vitamin B₁₂)

Vitamin B₁₂ (cyanocobalamin) supplementation to boys or normal young men did not change half-mile run times,[218] grip strength, heart rate recovery, maximal cycle ergometer times,[219] VO₂max, and other standard strength tests.[220] Evidence for a subjective "tonic" effect on patients complaining of "tiredness" was found for hydroxocobalamin (B₁₂) injections in a double-blind crossover study.[221] Relation of these finding to athletes may explain the popularity of B₁₂ injections and B₁₂ supplements. Currently, the primary, coenzymatic form of

B_{12}, known as cobamamide, Dibencozide™ or 5,6-dimethyl-benzimidazolyl cobamide coenzyme[222] has become a popular supplement among weightlifters.[223,224] Promotional literature contains a favorable comparison of cobamamide with anabolic steroids as an anabolic agent. What is not generally explained is that the study referred to was performed with 35 young children with growth deficiencies, osteoporosis, or hypoproteinemia.[225] Other supporting evidence of B_{12} as an "anabolic agent" is found in European pharmacopeias, but no studies on athletes are found.

6. Folates

Treatment of 10 nonanemic, folate-deficient, female marathon runners with 5 mg/d of folic acid for 11 weeks raised serum folate levels three- to four-fold, while serum levels of a placebo group decreased significantly.[226] However, VO_2max, maximal treadmill performance, heart rates, and blood lactate levels did not change in placebo- or folate-supplemented subjects. Higher serum folate levels were not associated with enhanced performance.

7. Pantothenate (Vitamin B_5)

Pantothenate (1 g daily for 2 weeks) has been shown to be ineffective in changing treadmill run times to exhaustion or blood glucose levels,[227] while another study administered 2 g daily for 2 weeks to trained distance runners and found decreases in blood lactate and oxygen consumption during prolonged strenuous cycling.[228]

8. B-Complex Vitamin Mixtures

Supplementation with mixtures of B-complex vitamins has yielded ambiguous results on human physical performance. Early reports found no significant effects on exhaustive exercise,[198,201,204,229] but vitamin B_{12} was not part of the complexes, and vitamin B_6 was present in only one study. A recent report with double-blind experimental design did not find a change in treadmill endurance capacity after 6 weeks with supplementation.[1] However, one early study reported an improvement of efficiency in tasks involving physical effort and coordination after niacin, riboflavin, thiamine, and vitamin C supplementation.[196] Another report utilizing a double-blind design found a significant reduction of fatigue in high school males running in a hot environment.[230] This study utilized higher daily doses of thiamine (100 g) and pantothenate (30 mg) than any other study, as illustrated in Table 2.

A review by Williams confirmed that more research on megadoses of vitamins and athletic performances is needed.[200] Also stated by Williams was the ability of B complex vitamins to "...give a better control of fine motor control..."[200] Another study by Bonke and Nickel administered 300 mg thiamine, 600 mg pyridoxine, and 600 mcg B12 daily for 8 weeks to pentathlete marksmen in a double-blind study.[231] Less muscle tremor, better control of fine muscles, and firing accuracy were significantly improved in the supplemented group.[231] Another double-blind study examined functional

TABLE 2
Comparative Daily Doses, Administration Schedules, and Ergogenic Effects of Controlled Human Studies on B Vitamin Supplements

Investigator	Year	B₁ (mg)	B₂ (mg)	Niacin (mg)	B₆ (mg)	B₁₂ (μg)	Panto. (μg)	Folate (mg)	C (mg)	Length of admin.	Conc.[a]	Ref.
Karpovich	(1942)	5								7 d	−	202
Foltz	(1942)	25[b]								acute[c]	−	201
Knippel	(1986)	900								3 d	+	206
Foltz	(1942)									acute	−	201
Haralambie	(1976)		10[b]							acute	+	207
Frankau	(1943)		10	50–200						acute	+	196
Jenkins	(1965)			300						acute	−[d]	209
Carlson	(1963)			500						acute	−[d]	208
Bergstrom	(1969)			500						acute	+[d]	211
Norris	(1978)			600						acute	−[d]	210
Lawrence	(1974)				51					6 mo	−	214
Marconi	(1982)				985[e]					30 d	−	218, 219
Montoye	(1955)			2000						7 wk	−	220
Tih-May-Than	(1978)					50				6 wk	−	227
Nice	(1984)					1000	1000			14 d	−	228
Litoff	(1985)						2000			14 d	−	226
Matter	(1987)		2		2			500	70	11 wk	+	233
Buzina[f]	(1982)		5	50					100	3 mo	+	196
Frankau	(1943)		5	100						4 d	+	205
Henschel	(1944)		10		60					3 d	−	231
Boncke	(1989)	90			60	120				8 wk	+	231
Boncke	(1989)	300			600	600				8 wk	+	231
Foltz	(1942)	15[b]	1.7[b]	50[b]	5[b]					acute	−	201
van der Beek	(1988)[g]	2.5	4	50[b]	4				100	8 wk	−	232

Simonson	(1942)	6	8	80	0.03	–	–	±	195	6 wk
Read	(1983)	5	5	25	2	0.5	12.5	–	1	acute
Keys	(1942)	5–17	10	100	10–100	20	200	–	203	4–6 wk
Early	(1969)	100	8	100	5	25000	30	+	230	acute

a Conclusion of study results: + indicates improved physiological change or enhanced performance. – indicates no effect on performance or physiological variables.
All doses are oral unless otherwise indicated.
b Intravenous administration.
c Acute signifies administration 0–2 h before exercise.
d Performance and/or physiological measurements showed detrimental changes.
e Actual administration was 16 mg/kg with a mean bodyweight of 61.6 ± 1.6 (S.E.M.) kg, for an average dose of 985 mg/d.
f Up to one-third of subjects showed clinical or biochemical symptoms of deficiencies for supplemented vitamins. This fact may mean observed benefits were due to repletion of deficiencies, which are known to decrease performance.
g Supplement included two times RDA amounts of vitamins A, D, E, B12, folate, biotin, niacinamide, and pantothenate to both the control and experimental groups.

performance of 12 subjects consuming a diet deficient in thiamine, riboflavin, and vitamins B6 and C (no more than 32.5% of RDA) for 8 weeks.[232] Eleven control subjects were fed the same diet with supplementation of twice the RDA for deficient vitamins. All subjects consumed supplements that supplied twice the RDA of other vitamins and adequate minerals and trace elements. No differences between groups were seen for physical activity monitors, submaximal performance, or mental performance (although the deficient group illustrated more errors with faster reactions). VO_2max, maximal workload, and blood lactate levels of control subjects did not change but did deteriorate for deficient subjects. Biochemical markers of vitamin status reflected a vitamin-deficient state for vitamins B1, B2, and B6 for deficient subjects and no changes for supplemented control subjects. This study is important because it showed that doses of B vitamins at twice the RDA do not influence body vitamin status, which correlates with lack of an ergogenic effect, similar to results of other studies using low doses of B vitamins (see Table 2).[1,195,198,200–205,229] Also, selection of common dietary foods may lead to vitamin deficiencies that adversely affect performance in 3 to 6 weeks.

In contrast, a European study found a small but significant increase in VO_2max after 80 schoolchildren, aged 12 to 15 years were given supplements containing 2 mg riboflavin, 2 mg pyridoxine, and 70 mg vitamin C.[233] However, up to 34% of these schoolchildren exhibited biochemical deficiencies of one or more of the supplemented vitamins. Whether the increase in performance was due to correction of deficiencies or ergogenic effects in nondeficient subjects was unknown.

A novel B-vitamin complex, α-ketoglutarate-pyridoxine (PAK), has been hypothesized to provide citric acid cycle intermediates, resulting in higher muscle ATP levels during heavy exercise.[214] Oral administration of PAK to 20 trained males (VO_2max = 58 ml/kg/min) was investigated.[214] Subjects ran an average of 10 to 15 km daily. Supplemented subjects received 30 mg/kg body weight (approximately 1850 mg/d) of PAK daily for 30 d. Measurements of VO_2max and anaerobic metabolism were performed before and after the supplement period. A significant increase in VO_2max (6%) was found for PAK users compared to an unsupplemented control period. Placebo users did not exhibit an increase in VO_2max compared to a control period. PAK did not influence the half-time of the VO_2 on-or-off responses. A decrease in lactate accumulation following a supramaximal treadmill run was exhibited after PAK supplementation, but not after supplementation with placebo, pyridoxine alone, or α-ketoglutarate alone. The authors proposed that increased transport of pyridoxine and α-ketoglutarate into mitochondria by PAK could account for the observed results.[214]

Effects of biotin, inositol, or p-aminobenzoic acid (PABA) on human exercise performance have not been reported. Some of these substances have been components of multiple mixtures which will be discussed in another section.

9. Summary and Guidelines

In summary, if no deficiencies exist, low to moderate doses (1 to 5 times RDA amounts) of supplemental B vitamins do not appear to enhance performance, and high doses of niacin may reduce performance. Upon closer examination, it is obvious that research on ergogenic effects of B vitamins is incomplete. First, very few studies examined megadoses (greater than 1000% RDA) of single or multiple B vitamins given before exercise or for more extended time periods. Those that did found significant improvements in physical performance.[228,230,231] This suggests that proper dose response studies have not been performed. Also, the differences between chronic and acute administration schedules have not been compared adequately. In addition, combined megadoses of each B vitamin listed in Table 2 have not been analyzed, except in two reports with only three and six components, both of which found some ergogenic properties.[230,231]

Another variable not yet considered in athletic performance is use of different forms of vitamins shown to have greatly increased absorption or metabolic effects over the traditional forms. Congeners of thiamine and pantothenic acid are available commercially and show properties that theoretically appear to be attractive to athletes. Allithiamines are lipid-soluble thiamine derivatives that exhibit dramatically increased absorption into tissue and therapeutic efficacy over thiamine hydrochloride or mononitrate.[234–236] Long-term safety and biopotency in humans after large oral doses (50 mg/d) have been reported.[236] A current review reiterated the increased efficacy of fat-soluble thiamine congeners (allithiamines) over water-soluble thiamines for clinical conditions, although exercise performance had still not been studied.[237]

Pantethine (the disulfide of pantetheine) consists of pantothenate bound to cysteamine and is a direct precursor of coenzyme A. Coenzyme A levels in perfused rat livers after pantethine administration were significantly elevated compared to control or pantothenate perfusion.[238] Pantethine administration has been shown to have antiarrhythmic actions on rodent and canine hearts, with increases in intracellular ATP hypothesized to account for these actions.[239–241] Pantethine supplementation significantly reduces elevated blood lipids and increases HDL cholesterol and apolipoprotein A in human subjects,[242–245] with a postulated mechanism of accelerated coenzyme A synthesis. Oral pantetheine administration (1 g/d) increased peak serum pantothenate levels tenfold.[246] Possible effects of increased pantothenate levels arising from pantetheine administration on athletes have not been reported, however. Since large doses of thiamine and pantothenate appeared to have ergogenic properties (see Table 2),[206,228,230] studies using congeners of these two vitamins to explore potential ergogenic effects are indicated.

Use of pyridoxal-5-phosphate, the coenzymatic form of vitamin B_6, is currently in vogue, especially among strength athletes consuming large amounts of dietary protein. There is little evidence to support advantages of oral supplementation of phosphorylated forms of vitamins over nonphosphorylated forms, however.

In conclusion, a need for further studies with particular attention to dose response, megadoses, potential toxicities of pyridoxine, a full complement of B vitamins, time of administration, and use of analogs is indicated. In particular, large doses of thiamine and pantothenate appear to have potential ergogenic effects, probably due to their key roles in cellular energy production. Another concept that concerns B vitamin supplementation is effects on nervous system function. Also, a link between clinically hidden cobalamin deficiencies and mood needs further exploration. A potential for reduction of depression, and thus, a more positive mental attitude, from cobalamin supplementation may explain the popularity of vitamin B_{12} supplements and injections.

Definitive studies on the issue of B vitamin supplementation and exercise performance have not been completed. With excessive market abundance, relative inexpensiveness, proven safety of large doses (if not taken chronically), and known mechanisms of action, further study of B vitamin effects on exercise performance would greatly aid athletes in general, regardless of outcome.

At this time, no definitive guidelines on B vitamin supplementation for purposes of enhanced performance are available, except for the avoidance of large doses of niacin (>300 mg per dose) before endurance exercise. If diet is proven or strongly suspected to be insufficient for B vitamins, a supplement containing 100% of the USRDA for B vitamins should prevent potential decreases in performance caused by deficiencies. Speculative guidelines for strenuous exercise would involve doses of 100 to 1000 mg/d for both thiamin and pantothenate. Another speculative guideline would be to include a supplement containing 50 to 100 mg (mcg for B_{12}) of each B vitamin for sports requiring a steady hand (archery, biathlon, target shooting, darts, baseball, race car driving). It is emphasized that the efficacy of speculative guidelines has not been conclusively confirmed.

B. VITAMIN C (ASCORBIC ACID)

This section will present a summary of results of vitamin C supplementation and human physical performance. Since its discovery in 1928, vitamin C (or ascorbic acid) has received much attention both scientifically and popularly. Widespread use, availability, and low cost have prompted numerous studies on human performance, with results that are confusing, confounding, contestable, confrontational, contentious, contradictory, and controversial. Nevertheless, a proposed mechanism of action being a protection or facilitation of oxidative reactions has been proposed.[247]

Early studies and many later studies almost always suffered from either a lack of controls, relatively low doses of vitamin C (less than 600 mg/d), nonstandard measurements of performance, or they provided no data, rendering results of these studies suspect.[192,196,200,203,205,247–278] No adequately controlled studies using less than 500 mg/d of vitamin C revealed ergogenic effects. Ten studies utilizing relatively high doses of vitamin C (greater than 600 mg/d or 1000% of USRDA), and adequate controls reveal conflicting conclusions.

Efficiency of submaximal work at a constant load of 120 watts (W) for 20 min was significantly increased after 5 d of supplementation with 1 g vitamin

C daily.[279] Another study of efficiency during a 5-min step test showed an increase in efficiency of 25% and significant reductions in total energy cost, oxygen debt, oxygen consumption, pulmonary ventilation, and heart rate.[280] These benefits may be confounded owing to nonrandomization of the order of administration, possibly allowing a training effect to occur.

Twelve weeks of daily 1 g doses of vitamin C did not affect performance of a 12-min walk/run test in 112 U.S. Air Force officers compared to a placebo group of 100 officers, suggesting vitamin C did not alter endurance performance.[281] In another study, 2 g of vitamin C were given daily to both smokers and nonsmokers for 5 d.[282] No effects of vitamin C were seen for respiratory adjustment and oxygen utilization before, during, or after exercise for smokers and nonsmokers.

Thirteen athletes were tested for metabolic changes, total performed work to exhaustion, and PWC 170 after 2 weeks of placebo administration and then after 2 weeks of supplementation with 1 g of vitamin C once daily in the morning.[283] Vitamin C supplementation did not affect total performed work, but led to a significant increase in PWC 170 with a lower heart rate. Excretion rate of vanillylmandelic acid was significantly increased by vitamin C, suggesting a higher turnover rate of catecholamines. Blood glucose levels were slightly but significantly decreased during exercise compared to the placebo period, while plasma-FFA levels were increased during exercise to a significantly greater extent in the supplemental period compared to the placebo period. The authors concluded that vitamin C caused beneficial changes in cardiovascular and metabolic parameters but not in endurance performance.[283]

Field tests of sprinting, long-distance running, and the Harvard Step test on track athletes showed no observed effects of vitamin C supplementation with 0 to 1 g daily for several weeks.[284] Ten athletes were tested for ventilation, heart rate, respiratory quotient, and blood lactate during cycle ergometry exercise at 60% VO₂max.[198] Measurements were made before and after a 7-d period of diet containing no vitamin C, and after 7 d of supplementation with 3 g of vitamin C daily. The only significant difference after vitamin C supplementation was a decrease in lactate levels.

Maximal cycle ergometer workloads (anaerobic exercise) were not affected 2 h after ingestion of 0.5 to 2.0 g of vitamin C.[285] Thirty-three sedentary young males participated in a double-blind study measuring VO₂max and anaerobic capacity on cycle ergometers.[286] Sixteen subjects received 1 g of vitamin C for 21 d. No effects of vitamin C on aerobic or anaerobic capacities were seen. A double-blind crossover study with 15 young males measured maximum grip strength and muscular endurance by a hand dynamometer.[287] Subjects received 600 mg vitamin C or a placebo 4 h before testing. Vitamin C supplementation did not exhibit significant differences from placebo values.

A recent double-blind study compared the effects of a low dose (500 mg) of vitamin C to a high dose (2000 mg).[288] Both acute (4 h prior to testing) and chronic (supplementation for 1 week) modes of administration for each dose were tested. Measurements of muscular strength (quadriceps and pectoral muscles), muscular endurance, and VO₂max were determined on 24 subjects.

Acute dosing with 500 mg vitamin C led to significantly improved quadriceps strength and a significantly reduced VO_2max, with no effect on quadriceps endurance or pectoral strength or endurance. Acute dosing with 2000 mg vitamin C produced no significant changes in VO_2max or muscular strength and endurance. Chronic supplementation with 500 mg vitamin C for 7 d resulted in significantly increased quadriceps and pectoral muscle strength, but reduced muscular endurance (quadriceps and pectoral) and significantly reduced VO_2max. Chronic supplementation with 2000 mg vitamin C for 7 d resulted in a significantly reduced VO_2 only. When compared to acute high doses, chronic high doses led to improved muscular endurance and lower VO_2max. The mixed results of this study may explain some of the contradictory results seen in other reports concerning the effects of vitamin C on human performance.

A positive correlation between plasma vitamin C levels under 1.0 mg/dl and VO_2max was found in boys aged 12 to 15 years.[289] Levels of higher than 1.0 mg/dl did not produce increases in VO_2max. This plasma level corresponded to a daily vitamin C intake of 80 mg.

1. Summary and Guidelines

In summary, most studies of vitamin C and physical performance are subject to experimental errors or administered doses near average daily intakes. Those studies that did incorporate adequate controls, measurements, and doses reveal ambiguous results (see Table 3). Several of these studies may have suffered from a training effect because order of administration of placebo and vitamin C was not randomized.[198,281,282,284,285] Also, no studies have measured performance at true body saturation of vitamin C at bowel tolerance doses (usually 10 g or more per day). A double-blind study using these doses would be most difficult, however.

One possible mechanism of action for vitamin C is as an antioxidant. Antioxidant effects of vitamin C can mimic superoxide dismutase activity in organisms.[290] The fat-soluble derivative of vitamin C (ascorbyl palmitate) has not been tested on exercised animals or subjects. Animal studies on vitamin C must take into account that humans and guinea pigs are the only mammalian models available that do not synthesize vitamin C endogenously.[291] Only a few studies on humans have measured metabolic changes pertinent to exercise, such as glucose, FFA, lactate, antioxidant status, etc. Those studies reporting measurements have found significant effects of vitamin C which suggest glycogen-sparing actions (see Table 3).

In conclusion, chronic use of vitamin C may not be associated with improvements in aerobic or anaerobic endurance, while a consensus on acute administration has not been reached. Obviously, further detailed research, employing double-blind controls with randomized crossover designs and large acute doses of vitamin C with evaluation of metabolic, hormonal, antioxidant, and performance changes, is needed to more fully evaluate ergogenic effects of vitamin C.

TABLE 3
Vitamin C Dose-Response and Ergogenic Effects

Investigator	Year	Ref.	Dose (g)	Length of adm.		Ergogenic effects[a]
Bender	(1975)	284	0 0–1 0	4 wk	( )	performance times for sprints and long-distance runs
Bramich	(1987)	288	0.5	acute	(+)	↑ quadriceps strength
					(–)	↓ VO$_2$max
					( )	muscular endurance
Bramich	(1987)	288	0.5	7 d	(+)	↑ muscular strength
					(–)	↓ muscular endurance & VO$_2$max
Inukai	(1977)	285	0.5–2.0	acute	( )	maximal cycle ergometer workload
Keith	(1983)	287	0.6	acute	( )	maximal grip strength or endurance
Hoogerweif	(1963)	279	1.0	5 d	(+)	↑ efficiency of submaximal work
Spioch	(1966)	280	1 0		(+)	↑ efficiency, ↓ energy cost, O$_2$ debt, O$_2$ consumption, pulmonary ventilation, heart rate
Gey	(1970)	281	1 0	4 wk	( )	endurance performance (U.S. Air Force walk/run test)
Howald	(1975)	283	1.0	2 wk	(+)	↑ peak work capacity at 170 W; ↓ heart rate, catecholamine excretion, exercise glucose
					( )	total work performed
Keren	(1980)	286	1 0	3 wk	( )	aerobic or anaerobic capacity
Bailey	(1970)	282	2.0	5 d	( )	O$_2$ utilization, respiratory effects, exercise plasma free fatty acid levels
Bramich	(1987)	288	2.0	acute	( )	↓ VO$_2$max, muscular strength and endurance
Bramich	(1987)	288	2 0	7 d	(–)	↓ VO$_2$ max
					( )	muscular strength or endurance
Keys	(1943)	198	3 0	7 d	(+)	↓ lactate levels
					( )	ventilation, heart rate, respiratory quotient

[a] (+) = beneficial ergogenic response (improved performance or physiological parameter);
(–) = detrimental ergogenic response (decreased performance or physiological parameter);
( ) = no effect

Guidelines for effective supplementation with vitamin C would be premature at this time. Daily doses of 0.5 to 2.0 g appear to be adequately safe for long-term use in most individuals. Except as a component of antioxidant mixtures (see later section on antioxidants), ergogenic effects of vitamin C are inconsistent.

C. FAT-SOLUBLE VITAMINS

1. Vitamin A (Retinols) and β-Carotene

Retinol (vitamin A) is vital for epithelial cell function.[292] It has been hypothesized that deficiencies in vitamin A may adversely affect sports that require visual acuity.[293] One report on the maximal endurance capacity of subjects on a vitamin A-deficient diet for 6 months noted no changes in endurance, although plasma vitamin A was not decreased, indicating a true deficient state was not reached.[294] The same report also noted no effects of vitamin A supplementation on endurance.[294] Thus, supplemental vitamin A appears to provide no benefit to physical performance.

Caution in preventing toxicity from overdoses of vitamin A is indicated, as toxicity has been seen after doses of 25,000 IU/d after many years of usage.[292,295] However, given the availability of supplements containing vitamin A in high doses (25,000 IU per unit) and given the large number of athletes consuming vitamin supplements,[199] only one case report of vitamin A intoxication in an athlete (an American soccer player) has been reported.[296] This demonstrates the superior safety record of unregulated vitamin supplementation as opposed to both unregulated and regulated pharmaceutical usage. For almost absolute safety where vitamin A (retinol or retinyl esters) supplementation is concerned, doses of 25,000 IU daily or less for nonpregnant women should not be exceeded unless under the advice of a physician.

β-carotene, a precursor of vitamin A, is also a quencher of singlet oxygen,[297] and thus has antioxidant properties. Conceivably, as with other antioxidants, a role in prevention of fatigue is possible, but no studies on effects of exercise performance in humans or animals after β-carotene supplementation was found (see later section on antioxidants for results from combinations including β-carotene). One report indicated serum β-carotene levels between amenorrheic and ovulatory groups of female long-distance runners were not different,[298] suggesting that β-carotene levels are not changed significantly by exercise. Unlike retinol, high doses of β-carotene are quite safe,[292,299,300] and conversion of β-carotene to retinol only occurs when retinol is deficient.[292,299]

2. Vitamin D (Calciferols)

Vitamin D is actually a series of sterols with hormone-like activity promoting bone calcification and intestinal calcium absorption.[301] Deficiencies in the U.S. are exceedingly rare, while huge overdoses are toxic,[301] especially in combination with UV light exposure (sunlight). Although no rationale for vitamin D supplementation is apparent, two studies have reported the effects on performance. Oral administration of cholecalciferol (vitamin D_3) to six subjects did not improve cycle ergometer performance.[302] Another report measured submaximal performance by the PWC-170 test on 60 school children aged 10 to 11 years.[303] Doses of 1600 IU (400 IU is the RDA) over long periods of time and even single doses of 400,000 IU did not improve performance. No subsequent reports have been found concerning the effects of vitamin D supplementation on exercise performance in normal subjects or athletes. Thus, vitamin D supplementation appears to be ineffective as an ergogenic aid.

3. Vitamin E (Tocopherols)

Presentation of possible mechanisms of ergogenic action and results of exercise performance trials will be presented in this section. Vitamin E (tocopherol) has well-known antioxidant functions protecting biomembranes from free radical damage.[304,305] Vitamin E supplementation was originally hypothesized to benefit athletic performance based on findings in tocopherol-deficient animals. Increased urinary excretion of creatine and phosphate, increased oxidation of polyunsaturated fatty acids, decreased ATP production, and increased levels of lactate and pyruvate, leading to a form of muscular dystrophy seen in deficient animals, prompted studies on the effects of supplemental vitamin E.[306] Adding to confusion among researchers was the initial use of wheat germ oil as a source of vitamin E. Subsequent studies confirmed that factors in wheat germ oil other than vitamin E accounted for observed ergogenic effects.[307]

Upon inspection of reports of vitamin E supplementation on human physical performance,[198,199,306-320] only three reports are published in major journals,[309,314,320] while two other reports are unpublished theses.[310,313] Most of these studies were hampered by lack of controls, reliance on anecdotal data, or crude performance measurements, thus relegating conclusions to be suggestive in nature.[198,199] However, vitamin E supplementation was shown to lower blood lactate levels after exercise compared to controls in one study.[306] Another study measured decreases in lipid peroxidation products (pentane) formed by 60 min of graded cycle exercise after supplementation with 1200 IU of vitamin E for 2 weeks, although pulmonary function was unchanged.[321] A double-blind placebo-controlled crossover study utilizing 800 IU vitamin E daily for 4 weeks in 8 subjects running at 80% VO_2max for 30 min found that post-exercise lipid hydroperoxide values were increased during the placebo period, but not during vitamin E supplementation.[322] Thus, vitamin E usage reduced oxidative damage induced by high intensity exercise. Likewise, effects of vitamin E supplementation (300 mg/d for 4 weeks) on serum lipid peroxide levels after acute exhaustive exercise in male college students was examined.[323] Exhaustive exercise led to significant increases in serum lipid peroxides and considerable leakage of enzymes from muscles. After supplementation with vitamin E, serum lipid peroxides decreased, and leakage of enzymes was lower.

Supplementation of 400 mg/d of vitamin E to mountain climbers at high altitudes for 4 weeks completely prevented the loss in anaerobic threshold seen in unsupplemented control subjects.[320] Breath pentane exhalation increased

104% in control subjects, but decreased 3.0% in supplemented climbers. It was concluded that vitamin E supplementation had a beneficial effect on physical performance and tissue protection at high altitude.[320] The only other well-controlled study to show a significant increase in performance caused by vitamin E utilized subjects at altitudes of 5000 and 15,000 ft.[313] Increased VO_2max (9 and 42%), decreased submaximal exercise oxygen uptake (0 and 7.1%) and reduced oxygen debt (16.5 and 20.1%) were reported for 12 subjects in a double-blind crossover study. These findings are consistent with known functions of vitamin E and with animal studies about vitamin E and altitude survival.[324-327]

Eight studies have shown no significant differences in performance after vitamin E supplementation.[198,213,306,321,328-334] In general, these studies were adequately controlled and some used doses of 1200 to 1600 IU vitamin E per day. However, five studies utilized swimmers as subjects[213,328-333] and another study did not include measurements that would reflect vitamin E functions.[335] The other two studies did not find changes in pulmonary function,[321] or in VO_2max.[335] Measurements in swimmers included VO_2max, muscular strength, ECG readings, run and swim times, or other physical tasks. Also, one report found no differences in blood lactate levels post-exercise between control and vitamin E-supplemented (900 IU/d for 6 months) groups.[328] Serum creatine kinase levels after exercise of trained or untrained muscle groups were not changed by 6 weeks of vitamin E supplementation at 447 IU/d of d-α-tocopheryl acetate.[336] Recently, prisoners performing "hard physical labor" such as coal shoveling were made deficient in vitamin E.[337] They showed no decreases in performance, even though blood levels of vitamin E were decreased by one-half. One other report did notice significant differences in respiratory parameters between those given a placebo and those treated with 800 or 1600 IU dl-α-tocopherol on short-term exposure to ozone,[338] and vitamin E supplementation was recommended for athletes participating in the 1984 Summer Olympic games at Los Angeles.[339]

It is interesting to note the lack of research on supplemental vitamin E administration and human athletic performance since 1978 until recently, even though a need for further research on performance at high altitudes was stated repeatedly.[331,332] Recent animal studies confirm that vitamin E can possess ergogenic effects (increased swimming time from 276 to 415 sec), based on antioxidant actions.[340] However, doses and length of administration of vitamin E in human studies is most likely insufficient to replicate animal findings. Other areas of vitamin E application which research has not addressed include scuba diving and other sports in hypoxic or hyperbaric settings.

The form of vitamin E utilized in studies was not specified in several reports.[328,329] Absorption differences between forms are not trivial and may account for lack of effects by some studies, since d-α-tocopherol produces much higher plasma (40%) and erythrocyte (300%) levels than synthetic d,l-α-tocopherol acetate.[341-343] In addition, absorption of vitamin E from dry or oily forms is limited, especially at higher doses,[342] while absorption of properly emulsified vitamin E preparations may further increase absorption.[344,345]

Overall, however, the use of vitamin E as an ergogenic aid is not supported, except at high altitudes. Further research on specific applications is indicated. Finally, vitamin E may serve as a protective agent against free-radical damage produced by exercise,[346] similar to protection seen in animal studies.[347–350] This finding may have health benefits after long-term usage.

Guidelines for effective use of vitamin E are 200 to 800 IU (mg)/d of d-α-tocopherol or mixed tocopherols (a combination of forms found in whole foodstuffs), preferable to dl- forms or esterified acetate or succinate forms. Mountain climbers, cross-country skiers, those who exercise at altitudes greater than 1.2 km, and those who exercise in cities with high levels of auto exhaust pollution are the groups with the best chance of ergogenic effects or protection from adverse effects by use of vitamin E.

4. Vitamin K (Menadiones and Phylloquinones)

Menadione (vitamin K) is involved in formation of blood clotting proteins and osteocalcin, important for bone health.[351] Deficiencies cause bruising and hemorrhaging, and are seen rarely after antibiotic or anticonvulsive therapy.[351] Normally, deficiencies are not seen in exercising populations, and as no rationale for ergogenic benefits from menadione supplementation is apparent, no studies have been performed.

Chapter 4

MICRONUTRIENT SUPPLEMENTATION AND ERGOGENESIS — METABOLIC INTERMEDIATES

I. ALKALINIZERS (BICARBONATE)

A. PH AND PERFORMANCE

Blood pH (normally 7.35 to 7.45) is tightly controlled by a bicarbonate buffer system even during exercise, when blood pH can drop to 7.0 and muscle pH from 7.0 to 6.4.[352-355] Lactic acid formed by anaerobic glycolysis is the primary acidifier during exercise.[354] Lowered pH inhibits phosphofructokinase, the rate-limiting step in glycolysis,[356,357] leading to fatigue. Thus, acidosis is one major factor causing fatigue during exercise.[354] This statement is further supported by numerous observations of decreased exercise performance after induced metabolic or respiratory acidosis.[358-367] Conversely, the hypothesis that metabolic alkalosis will increase the body's buffer reserve and thus delay fatigue has been tested repeatedly since the 1930s.

B. HUMAN STUDIES WITH BICARBONATE

Most early reports noted an increase in blood pH, postexercise blood lactate, oxygen debt, and/or performance during exhaustive treadmill or cycle exercises,[368-372] or improvement of race times (from 200 to 3200 m[359-373] after large doses of sodium bicarbonate (10 g) or mixtures of citrates and bicarbonate were given. When measured, physiological parameters supported the findings of increased performance, although a few studies were not adequately controlled or employed low subject numbers. Several studies did not find increased performance after alkalosis, but doses or administration schedules did not compare to previous studies.[374-377]

Recent experiments have examined the effects of alkalosis induced by bicarbonate on both anaerobic and aerobic exercise. In those studies that examined anaerobic, short-term exercise performance times after large doses of bicarbonate (0.2 to 0.3 g/kg body weight) were given 1 to 3 h before exercise, a majority have reported increased times to fatigue and/or reduced perception of fatigue, lowered plasma levels of enzymes released after muscular damage (CPK, GOT, GPT, OCT, aldolase), with greater blood lactate, pH, base excess and bicarbonate levels.[362,363,370,378-399]

Other studies did not find increases in performance,[366,367,377,378,382,400-411] even though blood pH and lactate values were changed significantly by alkaline loading.[367,378,403-406] Possibly, performance results were not enhanced due to insufficient exercise time,[367,378,403-406] variability in subject training or mechanical efficiency,[382,407] methodological difficulties,[402] or insufficient dose.[378,403,411] Some studies reported few details,[400,403] while other studies did not find significant changes in blood pH, lactate, or performance.[367,378] Bicarbonate loading had no effect on time to exhaustion in a submaximal exercise test lasting over 30 min.[412]

C. SUMMARY AND GUIDELINES

Overall, a consensus of literature indicates that bicarbonate loading can increase performance time for short-term intense exercise, provided the exercise bouts are repeated more than twice in a short period of time. A recent review stated that when exhaustive exercise lasted 1 to 7 min, bicarbonate loading showed beneficial ergogenic effects.[377]

Although excessive alkalosis theoretically has negative effects,[354] and performance with blood pH greater than 7.5 reportedly caused decreases in performance,[403] it appears that a mildly elevated blood pH of 7.4 to 7.5 at start of exercise is associated with increased anaerobic performance. Tolerance to lactate via increases in body-buffering capacity,[354,382,384,405] sparing of muscle glycogenolysis and creatine phosphate,[363,381] greater efflux of H^+ and lactate from muscle cells,[382,405] and possibly increased utilization of lactate as a fuel[354] are thought to contribute to the beneficial ergogenic effects of alkaline loading.

Information regarding the use of alkalinizers other than bicarbonate is scarce. Citrate has been used, with or without bicarbonate, and trihydroxymethylaminomethane (TRIS) has also been used, but it is a potent diuretic. Caution with ingestion of large doses of sodium bicarbonate is necessary. Excessive doses have produced nausea, vomiting, flatulence, diarrhea, and even muscle cramps.[355,362] Also, determination of urine pH (a very simple task) is sufficient to detect athletes who use alkaline loading, although no sports governing agency yet considers this practice to be doping.

In conclusion, alkaline loading will not affect VO_2max, heart rate, or strength, but has been shown to consistently improve maximal performance during repeated short-term anaerobic exercise tasks for trained subjects. Interestingly, no studies employing weight lifters (a repeated anaerobic task) have been reported. Findings of decreased fatigue in weight lifters would further confirm the concept of alkalosis as an ergogenic aid. Studies employing potassium bicarbonate or mixtures of sodium and potassium bicarbonate have not been described.

Sodium bicarbonate (baking soda) is a normal body component, readily available commercially, inexpensive, and currently used by thousands for minor medical problems, albeit at low doses. Guidelines for use of baking soda (bicarbonate) suggest that, for trained athletes engaged in exhaustive anaerobic events lasting between 1 and 7 min, bicarbonate loading (0.2 to 0.3 g/kg 30 to 60 min before the event) has a significant ergogenic effect.

II. ANTIOXIDANTS

A large array of compounds, ranging from single elements to large enzymatic complexes, are utilized to protect our bodies from oxidative, free radical-mediated damage. Collectively, these compounds are known as antioxidants. The field of free radical biology and medicine has become enormous, with spillover into exercise physiology. Exercise increases oxidative processes of muscle, leading to increased generation of free radicals[349,413–417] and lipid peroxides.[321,347–350,416–424] Subcellular damage, partly as a result of free-radical attack, has been observed after exercise.[416,417,422,425–429] Training induces higher levels of antioxidant enzymes superoxide dismutase (SOD) and catalase in both animal and human muscle tissue,[417,421,430–432] and reduces susceptibility of muscle to peroxidative damage.[421,433,434] Activities of antioxidant enzymes do not change immediately after an exercise bout, but the ratio of reduced/oxidized glutathione is decreased as much as fivefold, signifying that peroxidative stress has occurred.[435] It is also of interest to note the proinflammatory immunological changes that occur after exercise in humans.[435–437] These changes are an indication that leukocytes are activated, a process that produces oxygen-free radicals.[438–441]

A study measured swimming performance of mice after administration of synthetic spin-trappers (compounds that directly neutralize free radicals) N-t-butyl-α-phenyl-nitrone (PBN), 5,5-dimethyl-1-pirrolyn-N-oxide (DMPO), and α-4-pyridyl-1-oxide-N-t-butyl-nitrone (POBN).[340] Significantly improved swimming times (298 vs. 398, 493, and 555 sec after PBN, POBN and DMPO, respectively) were found, indicating that removal of free radicals would enhance aerobic performance.[340] Similarly, after rats were injected with the synthetic antioxidant BHT (20 mg/kg/d for 3 d), a 60% increase in maximum duration of treadmill running to exhaustion was found.[442] In addition, lipid peroxide levels in muscles were significantly lower at time of exhaustion after BHT supplementation.

A. HUMAN STUDIES

In 15 untrained humans given BHT (20 mg/kg per every 48 h for 15 d), exhalation of pentane (a marker for free radical damage to cell membranes) was greatly decreased after an exhaustive cycle ergometry test.[416]

Researchers at the University of California, Berkeley examined the effects of antioxidant supplementation on indices of muscle trauma and antioxidant status. Twenty-three moderately-trained runners were given a combination of β carotene (10 mg), vitamin E (800 IU), and vitamin C (1000 mg) daily for 3 to 4 weeks, and measurements were made before and after downhill treadmill running at 65% VO$_2$max.[443] Results showed significantly lower post-exercise levels of CPK and LDH, no increase in oxidized plasma glutathione (0 vs. 20%), a smaller decrease in reduced plasma glutathione (45 vs. 65%), and quicker recovery of altered antioxidant status after exercise. Thus, antioxidant supplementation enhanced antioxidant status and reduced indices of exercise-induced muscular trauma in humans.

As reported by Singh from a personal communication from Kantner, Nolte, and Holloszy, a double-blind, placebo-controlled study examined effects of supplementation with an antioxidant mixture consisting of vitamin C (1000 mg ascorbic acid), vitamin E (727 mg dl-α-tocopherol), and β-carotene (28 mg) on treadmill exercise that caused increased lipid peroxidation (elevated serum malondialdehyde and elevated breath pentane).[443a] Antioxidant supplementation significantly reduced both measures of free radical damage at rest and during exercise.

Eleven trained male subjects were tested by cycle ergometry (90 min at 65% VO_2max) before and after 28 d of supplementation with an antioxidant mixture (533 mg d-α-tocopherol, 1000 mg ascorbic acid, and 10 mg of β-carotene per day).[443b] Measurement of urinary 8-hydroxyguanosine was used as an indicator of free radical damage (RNA oxidation). Although levels of supplemented antioxidants were increased by 87% (vitamin E), 16% (vitamin C) and 480% (β-carotene), urinary output of 8-hydroxyguanosine was not affected by exercise before or after antioxidant supplementation. Perhaps more intense exercise is needed to exhibit exercise-induced oxidative damage to RNA in humans, and more or different antioxidants are needed to decrease measures of RNA oxidation.

Supplementation with 400 IU vitamin E and 500 mg of vitamin C daily for 6 months led to stimulation of T-cell mitogenesis and enhanced prostaglandin E synthesis by stimulated lymphocytes in both fit and sedentary subjects.[444] Fit subjects had higher mitogenesis than sedentary subjects. The authors concluded that physical conditioning and vitamin supplementation can stimulate cellular immune function in adults.

Thus, limited data on supplementation with synthetic antioxidants and mixtures of vitamin antioxidants support the hypothesis that damage from free radical mechanisms induced by exercise can be greatly alleviated. Whether this will have effects on exercise performance is not yet known, and requires further research.

B. SUMMARY AND GUIDELINES

Supplements containing SOD and catalase are being marketed specifically for athletes. Claims include increased endurance and well-being resulting from decreased levels of free-radical damage, especially to mitochondrial membranes. Upon analysis of products, actual enzyme contents per tablet varied from 0 to 18,590 McCord-Fridovich units for SOD and 0 to 22,990 Beer-Sizer units for catalase.[445] In addition, while absorption of therapeutic amounts of intact, active proteases through the gastrointestinal (GI) tract has been consistently documented,[446-453] the absorption of oral SOD has not been confirmed in animals,[454,455] although definitive studies have not been reported. Plant catalases (e.g., horseradish peroxidase) have been documented to cross the GI tract in animals,[456-458] and even to cross the blood-brain barrier in humans after oral administration.[459] However, objective reports on effects of oral antioxidant enzyme supplementation on athletes are lacking. Such testing is feasible, given a postulated mechanism of action, availability of supplements, and well-characterized testing methods for both peroxidative damage and antioxidant enzymes.

Guidelines on use of antioxidant mixtures are still premature in regard to enhancement of exercise performance. However, based on research with vitamin E and an extensive body of literature outside the scope of this book concerning protection from free radical damage and potential long-term health benefits from supplementation with antioxidants, those who exercise at high altitudes, in polluted air, or with frequent time zone changes may show actual enhancement of performance. In addition, any person may benefit from the long-term protective benefits of antioxidant supplementation. Antioxidant supplementation can be thought of as artificially providing the effects of exercise training, since both practices increase endogenous tissue levels of antioxidants and offer long-term health benefits. Speculative doses of an antioxidant mixture include 200 to 800 IU/d of vitamin E (preferably as d-α-tocopherols or mixed tocopherols), 15,000 to 50,000 IU/d of β-carotene, 0.5 to 2.0 g/d of vitamin C (ascorbate), and 100 to 250 μg of selenium (preferably as selenite).

III. ASPARTATE SALTS

A. MECHANISMS OF ACTION

The dispensable dicarboxylic amino acid, aspartic acid, is also a metabolic intermediate in several biochemical pathways such as the tricarboxylic acid and urea cycles.[460] Amino acid salts were hypothesized as mineral transporters to subcellular sites, aiding in metabolism by replenishment of electrolytes.[461] For these reasons, monopotassium and monomagnesium DL-aspartate in equal amounts were studied by Laborit and co-workers.[462–464] They deduced that metabolic effects from the aspartate moiety contributed to decreased oxygen consumption. Meanwhile, Nieper indicated that intracellular transport of potassium and magnesium by aspartate salts corrected deficiencies and reduced hypoxia in human ischemic hearts.[461]

Using animals, two reports suggested that monopotassium- and monomagnesium-L-aspartates or potassium-L-aspartate improved rat swim times,[465,466] but these results were not confirmed in two other studies.[467,468] Increases in rat muscle aspartate, contractility, ATP, and phosphocreatine levels were seen after i.p. injection of D,L-, D-, and L-aspartate potassium salts.[469,470] These results were not duplicated after oral administration.[468] Differences between D- and L-asparate salts of potassium and magnesium on resynthesis of ATP after muscle work were noted, indicating possible differences in effects between L- and D,L-aspartate salts.[470]

B. HUMAN STUDIES

Potassium and magnesium L-aspartate salts have been used medically to treat fatigue in human subjects,[471,472] although benefits were disregarded since fatigue estimation was subjective.[473] As reported by Shaw,[472] Laborit and co-workers measured muscular fatigue by rheotome in 144 French Army athletes. Reduced fatigue was found in 89% of subjects after potassium- and magnesium DL-aspartate administration. Soon thereafter, two reports on the effects of 2 g daily of presumably potassium- and magnesium L-aspartate on various weightlifting exercises, grip strength, runs to exhaustion, and submaximal treadmill walking in 38 subjects showed no convincing effects.[474,475] However, three reports of increased times to exhaustion (23 to 50%) on cycle ergometers after administration of 7 or 13 g/d of potassium- and magnesium D,L-aspartate renewed interest in aspartates.[476-478] Glycogen-sparing effects, increases in cardiorespiratory functions, and increases in oxidation of fatty acids were hypothesized as mechanisms of action. A significant increase in treadmill performance was seen for untrained subjects, but not for trained subjects, after 2 g/d of potassium- and magnesium L-aspartate administration over a 2 week period.[479] Administration of 10 g of potassium-magnesium aspartate to 7 trained, competitive, male athletes in a double-blind, crossover study 24 h before testing found a significant increase in time to exhaustion (14%) for treadmill runs at 75% VO_2max.[480] Aspartate dosing decreased blood lactate levels and blood ammonia levels and increased serum FFA levels, compared to placebo runs. This study utilized a higher aspartate dose than other studies, suggesting a dose response or threshold effect for aspartates may be apparent. Importantly, consistent decreases in blood ammonia and glycogen sparing (suggested by increased serum FFA levels) rather than changes in lactate or glucose (which were not seen) correlate with proposed mechanisms of action for aspartates.[462-464,476-478]

Although these studies utilized single- or double-blind designs, criticisms of low sample numbers (four to eight per study) and possibly lack of control prompted further studies. Three studies utilized double-blind placebo with untreated control designs and found no effects on short-term exercise,[468] treadmill walking performance,[481] cycle ergometer performance to exhaustion,[482] or physiological parameters.[468,482] One study utilized 8.4 g/d of potassium- and magnesium D,L-aspartate,[468] but the other studies did not specify whether L- and D,L-aspartate was administered. Interestingly, all reports have studied only young males. No females or older subjects were studied. In addition, three of four studies with untrained subjects showed significant increases in performance, whereas four of six studies with trained subjects showed no significant increases. Surprisingly, only two studies measured blood ammonia levels, and both found a trend towards decreased ammonia levels after aspartate administration, which fits the hypothetical mechanism of action. For further results on the use of aspartates on reducing blood ammonia (one factor in fatigue sensation), consult the section specific to amino acid effects in this chapter.

C. SUMMARY AND GUIDELINES

In summary, it appears that acute administration of 7 g or more of potassium- and magnesium D,L-aspartate within 24 h to untrained subjects may improve long-term performance. Before this conclusion can be regarded as definitive, further tests with larger numbers of subjects (including females) and rigorous control designs are necessary. Trained subjects appear to derive no benefit from D,L- or L-aspartate salts in short- or long-term exercises, although testing of females is lacking to confirm this conclusion. No physiological measurements are available from studies showing improvements in performance; therefore, a mechanism of action is unproven. Theoretically, stabilization of cellular membranes by normalization of intracellular potassium- and magnesium concentrations,[461] detoxification of ammonia,[462,464] or increase in tricarboxylic acid-cycle flux[462,464] are potential mechanisms of action of aspartate salts.

Guidelines for use of aspartate salts are suggested for untrained subjects about to undergo exhaustive exercise in a single event. At least 7 g of a mixture of potassium- and magnesium-D,L-aspartates ingested in two to three doses during the 24 h period before an event is suggested.

IV. CARNITINE

A. MECHANISMS OF ACTION

L-Carnitine (β-hydroxy-[γ-N-trimethylammonia]-butyrate), was discovered in muscle tissue in 1905.[483] Carnitine is primarily involved with transporting long-chain fatty acids from cell cytosol into mitochondria.[484-488] Since long-chain fatty acids (acyl groups) are oxidized ("burned") in mitochondria, carnitine facilitates production of energy from fats. The enzymes coenzyme A:carnitine acyl transferase and carnitine translocase are necessary to form and move acylcarnitines into mitochondria and free carnitine out of mitochondria.[486] Another acyl transferase enzyme separates the carnitine and fatty acid inside mitochondria, where the fatty acid undergoes β-oxidation, producing acetyl groups to enter the tricarboxylic acid (TCA or Krebs) cycle.[486] Carnitine thus frees coenzyme A (CoA) molecules for use in the cytosol, increasing TCA cycle flux, and decreasing levels of acyl CoA molecules, which inhibit ATP transport and damage cell membranes at low concentrations.[486] By formation of acetyl carnitine inside of mitochondria, carnitine can act as a reservoir of acetyl groups, which can enter the TCA cycle at a later time.[486] Oxidation of branched-chain amino acids (BCAAs) is facilitated by carnitine, providing a link between protein catabolism and cellular energy production.[486] These carnitine actions stimulate metabolism of pyruvate by pyruvate dehydrogenase, decreasing lactate buildup. All these functions are of primal importance to exercising muscle, since aerobic endurance training relies heavily upon fatty acid oxidation. BCAA oxidation during exercise is now recognized as a small but significant energy source during exercise. Underscoring these functions is the finding that skeletal muscle contains 90% of total body carnitine in humans.[487]

Carnitine is synthesized endogenously from the amino acids lysine and methionine and thus is not classified as an essential vitamin for adult humans.[487] Dietary intake (primarily from animal foodstuffs) also occurs, although dietary carnitine from foods is a minor source (approximately 50 mg daily).[487] Carnitine is almost nonexistent in plants (except molds), but if strict vegetarians consume adequate lysine and methionine, deficiencies are probably not encountered.[488] Inherited deficiencies in carnitine synthesis or dependent enzymes have been identified and are associated with severe muscular weakness and exercise intolerance, but these cases are rare.[485,487,488,917]

B. HUMAN STUDIES
1. Carnitine Metabolism During Exercise
Carnitine exists in humans as free (unesterified) carnitine, and esterified carnitine (acylcarnitines), both of which make up total carnitine. Any length of fatty acid can be esterified to carnitine. The simplest esterified carnitine is acetylcarnitine (2 carbon chain length), and both short-chain (3 to 12 carbons) and long-chain (14 or more carbons) acylcarnitines are present. Levels of total carnitine, free carnitine, esterified carnitine and types of esterified carnitine can be measured in urine, plasma and tissue samples (muscle biopsies) of humans. When measurements of carnitine metabolites are made accompanying exercise in humans, certain patterns have been consistently and reproducibly observed.

Exercise of sufficient intensity and duration produces large decreases in plasma[486,490–492,501–503,916,918] and muscle[491,919–924] free carnitine levels. For example, after a 13-h cross-country ski race, muscle free carnitine levels from 18 skiers decreased by 20%.[924] Simultaneously, increases of plasma[486,490–493,501–503,916,923] and muscle[919–924] acylcarnitine levels are produced by exercise. For example, after 3 to 4 min of cycle ergometry at 90% VO_2max, muscle acetylcarnitine levels rose from 6.0 to 15.2 mmol/kg dry weight.[922] Urine output of short-chain acylcarnitines has been observed after strenuous training.[923,925]

Alterations in carnitine metabolism by exercise show a clear-cut dependence on intensity and workload.[920–922] Low intensity, submaximal exercise (50% of lactate threshold work load or 30 to 40% VO_2max) for durations between 3 to 60 min did not change levels of carnitine metabolites in muscle biopsies.[920–922] However, during and after exercise of higher intensities (60 to 90% VO_2max or work loads between lactate threshold and maximal work capacity), decreased free carnitine and increased acylcarnitines were seen in muscle biopsies.[920–922] Thus, carnitine metabolism (homeostasis) is affected primarily by strenuous exercise, and less by mild exercise. In other words, normal levels of carnitine in muscle are sufficient to provide enough fatty acids for mitochondrial energy production pathways during exercise of low intensity. However, strenuous exercise places a metabolic demand upon carnitine function. In these cases, it is hypothesized that exogenous carnitine may facilitate greater entry of fatty acids into mitochondria and/or other functions that result in greater or longer production of muscular energy. These findings on carnitine metabolism in exercising humans should be kept in mind when interpreting results of carnitine supplementation trials.

2. Carnitine Supplementation and Exercise
A review of studies on carnitine supplementation and physical performance found that 1 to 6 g/d of supplemental carnitine for periods up to 6 months consistently increased plasma levels of total carnitine with no apparent toxicity or ill effects.[916]

Marconi et al. administered 4 g/d L-carnitine for 2 weeks to 6 trained long-distance walkers in a randomized-crossover blind study.[493] Total, free-, and esterified carnitine levels in serum increased significantly after supplementation, suggesting uptake into tissue occurred. Maximal aerobic power (VO_2max) was increased slightly (6%) but significantly after carnitine supplementation. The authors indicated a lower acetyl CoA/CoA ratio caused by carnitine could stimulate pyruvate dehydrogenase, increasing the flux of the TCA cycle and thus improving VO_2max. Lactate accumulation during two types of supramaximal (anaerobic) work was not affected. Importantly, respiratory quotient values were unchanged, indicating the excess carnitine did not increase utilization of long-chain fatty acids. This observation confirmed reports that fat oxidation in trained athletes is not limited by factors that regulate lipid use (e.g., carnitine).[496]

A French study cited by Marconi claimed that 4.8 g of L-carnitine per day for 3 weeks doubled the duration of a submaximal (80% VO_2max) endurance exercise with a significant decrease in respiratory quotient.[493] No other details were available.

A study of 30 males and 20 females (well-trained) at the Sports Polyclinic in Bucharest, Romania, given 3 g/d carnitine for 21 d found significant increases in VO_2max (11%), less blood lactate levels after exercise (7.9 vs. 9.9 mM) and lower plasma triglyceride levels.[926] Acute, intravenous administration of 1 g L-carnitine 60 min before exercise to 17 elite swimmers at the Sports Polyclinic in Bucharest in a double-blind, crossover trial was associated with significant changes compared to the placebo period in post-exercise values of plasma lactate, triglycerides, free fatty acids, and evoked muscular potential.[927] A series of 6 double-blind, placebo-controlled, randomized crossover trials at the Sports Polyclinic in Bucharest was conducted with 110 elite athletes (swimmers, rowers, canoers, weight lifters, and long-distance runners) to study effects on physiological parameters of carnitine supplementation.[928] Both acute, single doses of 1 g carnitine and daily doses of 1 to 3 g of carnitine for 3 weeks were administered. Significant changes after both acute and chronic carnitine administration, compared to placebo periods, were seen for post-exercise plasma lactate, triglycerides, free fatty acids, and evoked muscular potential. Changes in plasma and urine carnitine metabolites indicated increased free carnitine and post-exercise acetylcarnitine levels during supplemented periods. Results of this series of studies agree with the hypothesis that increased levels of free carnitine allow greater amounts of fatty acids to be utilized as an energy source during intense exercise.

An increase in peak anaerobic power in six healthy subjects was attributed to carnitine supplementation (4 g/d for 14 d).[916] This response was predicted, based on the known effects of carnitine on adenylate translocase in muscle mitochondria, resulting in increased resting levels of ATP and phosphocreatine in resting muscles.[916]

A double-blind, randomized crossover trial on 10 trained males for acute effects of carnitine supplementation on maximal exercise capacity was reported by Vecchiet.[929] Either placebo or 2 g L-carnitine were given 1 h before graded cycle ergometry to exhaustion. After a 72 h washout period, athletes were retested with the crossover agent. VO_2max and power output were significantly increased after L-carnitine supplementation. Plasma lactate, pulmonary ventilation, oxygen uptake, and carbon dioxide production were decreased after carnitine supplementation compared to similar exercise intensities from the placebo period. Changes in levels of plasma and urine carnitine metabolites, along with decreased levels of plasma lactate and pyruvate suggested that carnitine supplementation stimulated pyruvate dehydrogenase activity, diverting pyruvate from lactate to acetylcarnitine formation.[930] This suggests carnitine can serve as a type of buffer to decrease muscular lactate and conserve acetyl groups.[930] Thus, acute administration of carnitine was associated with more efficient exercise performance.

A double-blind, placebo-controlled, randomized crossover trial studied physiological parameters in 10 trained subjects after cycle ergometry for 45 min at 66% VO_2max.[931] The supplemented periods were 28 d of either placebo or 2 g/d of L-carnitine. A control exercise test was performed before the study period. No differences in measurements were observed between the control or placebo tests. However, after carnitine supplementation, a significantly lower respiratory quotient was seen, and nonsignificant trends towards higher values for oxygen uptake, heart rate, plasma glycerol and plasma free fatty acids were seen. These results suggest that carnitine supplementation may increase lipid utilization by muscles during exercise.

Effects of placebo or carnitine administration on physiological parameters following strenuous treadmill exercise at sea level or high-altitude (3500 m) conditions were studied in 7 healthy male subjects in a double-blind fashion.[932] No changes from carnitine supplementation at either altitude were observed for oxygen uptake, pulmonary ventilation, carbon dioxide output, heart rate, blood pressure, and serum levels of lactate, free fatty acids, glycerol, and glucose. However, significant decreases in respiratory quotient were found at each altitude. Thus, carnitine supplementation may improve lipid utilization during exercise under normoxic or hypoxic conditions.

Similarly, another study found decreases in post-exercise markers of free radical damage (plasma thiobarbituric acid reaction products) after carnitine or propionyl-L-carnitine supplementation.[933] This study indicates that free radical production in hypoxic (exercise) conditions can be antagonized by improved muscular utilization of fuel substrates.

Supplementation with 3.5 g/d of L-carnitine for 30 d to 6 trained subjects found improvements in carnitine metabolism (higher total, free- and esterified carnitine levels in plasma) after 60 min of cycle ergometry at 60% VO_2max.[501] Thirteen long-distance runners and eleven sprinters were given either a placebo or 1 g L-carnitine for 6 months.[923] Training lowered total and free muscle carnitine levels, due to an overflow of carnitine esters into the urine. Supplementation did not affect carnitine levels in blood, but muscle carnitine pools were stabilized, and in sprinters, the effects of training on loss of carnitine were prevented. Thus, long-term carnitine supplementation with a modest dose (compared to other studies) prevented exercise-induced loss of muscle carnitine into plasma and urine compartments. How these changes would affect exercise performance is unknown.

Two groups consisting of nineteen untrained subjects performing submaximal exercise were studied in two double-blind, crossover trials of carnitine supplementation (2 g/d carnitine for 14 or 28 d).[499] No changes in plasma levels of carnitine metabolites were measured, indicating that exercise was of low intensity. In Trial 1, a small improvement in submaximal performance was demonstrated by a decrease in the heart rate response to a work load corresponding to 50% VO$_2$max. However, there were no observable changes in VO$_2$max, or post-exercise lactate and β-hydroxybutyrate levels in plasma. Trial 2 did not reproduce the improvement in submaximal performance found in Trial 1, and no changes in VO$_2$max or heart rate were found. The contradictory results of this study are most likely due to the low intensity of exercise, which was insufficient to change carnitine homeostasis. The results suggest that carnitine supplementation has little effect on exercise of low intensity in untrained subjects.

Similar results (no change in submaximal VO$_2$) were found for 4 untrained males given 6 g/d carnitine for 10 d,[500] and 20 untrained males given 2 g/d carnitine for 28 d.[916] No significant effects on plasma lipid parameters (free fatty acids, glycerol, β-hydroxybutyrate) or mitochondrial enzymes were noted after carnitine supplementation (2 to 6 g/d) in athletes, from several previously unreported studies.[499,916]

Another double-blind crossover trial of carnitine supplementation (3 g/d for 5 d) to 7 trained male subjects exercising on a cycle ergometer for 120 min at 50% VO$_2$max measured physiological parameters related to carnitine functions.[503] Carnitine supplementation doubled plasma carnitine levels and resulted in lower heart rates (7 to 8%) during exercise. However, oxygen uptake, plasma free fatty acid levels, and uptake and turnover during exercise were unchanged by carnitine supplementation. Before carnitine supplementation, plasma levels of free carnitine decreased and esterified carnitine levels increased during exercise. The authors concluded that short-term carnitine supplementation did not influence muscle substrate utilization at rest or during low intensity, submaximal exercise.

Two recent abstracts describing two double-blind crossover studies of ten conditioned subjects found no significant effects after 4 weeks of L-carnitine supplementation on submaximal aerobic exercise.[507,508] Daily doses were 0.5 g, 4 to 8 times less than doses used in other studies showing ergogenic effects. Apparently, large daily doses of carnitine (>2 g/d), but not small doses (0.5 g/d) are needed before enhancement of aerobic exercise parameters is possible.

In a different type of performance study, adolescents receiving a supplement containing carnitine, vitamins, and sugars improved their ability to solve video-game tests.[509]

Because of potential effects for carnitine supplementation on enhancement of muscle energy production under ischemic conditions, and the need for heart muscle to derive most of its energy from oxidation of fatty acids, trials of carnitine supplementation in cardiovascular and pulmonary disease patients have been performed. Carnitine administration has been shown to improve exercise performance, ventilatory parameters, and metabolic responses to exercise for patients with Type A chronic respiratory insufficiency.[927,928] Numerous studies on effects of carnitine and propionylcarnitine supplementation (in addition to conventional therapies) to patients with angina pectoris, peripheral vascular disease or congestive heart failure all found significant improvements in exercise tolerance, exercise performance, total work output, cardiac function, blood lipid levels, and reductions in premature ventricular contractions, time to exertional pain and drug dosages.[512–516,934–939] One study was a multicenter trial with over 200 patients.[936] Another case of carnitine supplementation used in a disease state to enhance exercise performance is chronic hemodialysis. Some hemodialysis patients show a carnitine deficiency partly due to decreased kidney function (one vital step in carnitine synthesis occurs only in the kidney), and partly due to loss of carnitine during dialysis.[940] After intravenous replenishment of carnitine after dialysis sessions, improved exercise performance, increased VO_2max, decreased muscle cramps, decreased hypotension, increased muscle mass, decreased serum urea nitrogen, creatinine and phosphorus levels were observed during the intra-dialysis time period for 82 patients.[940] These medical situations represent extreme physiologic and metabolic conditions which may not apply to healthy individuals, but do reaffirm the known functions of carnitine. Therefore, use of carnitine in patients recovering from cardiovascular disease and told to initiate an exercise program may provide better compliance via better tolerance to exercise, and perhaps, performance.

C. SUMMARY AND GUIDELINES

Carnitine supplementation as an ergogenic aid has shown mixed results. For submaximal (low intensity) exercise, carnitine appears to have little or no value as a performance enhancer. However, both acute (immediately before exercise) and chronic (≥ 7 d of daily dosing) administration of L-carnitine in doses exceeding 1 g/d have been associated with some benefits in exercise metabolism and performance, when exercise has been sufficiently intense. Decreased heart rate for a given workload, improved VO_2max, improved use of lipids as a fuel, and stabilization of carnitine metabolite fluctuations during exercise have been observed in some, but not all, studies measuring these parameters. Five studies reported improvements in exercise performance after carnitine supplementation.[493,499,509,916,929] Two studies did not find changes in exercise performance.[499,502] One of these studies could not reproduce initial findings of increased submaximal exercise time in a second trial.[502] Thus, it is apparent that simply taking several grams per day of L-carnitine will not automatically improve exercise performance to a measurable extent. The fact that some studies have shown ergogenic effects means that carnitine may be effective under certain conditions, but not every condition. This knowledge, coupled with safety of large doses of carnitine[493] indicates that further research on the effects of carnitine supplementation on athletes is warranted. Determination of which exercise types, carnitine dosage and training status of individuals would produce reproducible ergogenic effects is a logical extension of current research.

Also, the combined effects of carnitine supplementation, exercise, and a low fat diet compared to exercise and low fat diet on body fat percentage of trained or untrained humans have not been studied. This would represent another practical application for carnitine supplementation, based on results to date.

A note of caution concerning the form of carnitine used for supplementation is needed. DL-Carnitine, which is much less expensive than L-carnitine, has been shown to cause muscle weakness in hemodialysis patients.[517,518] DL-Carnitine is now less available as a supplement for this reason. Only L-carnitine should be used in future studies to avoid the potential toxicity of the D-form of carnitine.

Of particular interest is the use of carnitine in patients with serious cardiovascular or pulmonary disease. Carnitine supplementation has never been associated with side effects or interactions with conventional therapies, and has reproducibly enhanced physical performance of these patients. Numerous studies suggest that carnitine supplementation may improve compliance of patients with exercise programs prescribed for them, or reduce painful symptoms of exertion. Of course, advice of a physician should be sought before a decision to administer carnitine in such patients is made.

Carnitine shows promise as an ergogenic aid for intense exercise. Guidelines for use of carnitine for trained athletes and patients initiating an exercise program while recovering from cardiovascular disease are at least 1 g/d for long time periods (6 months) or >3 g/d for shorter courses of supplementation (1 to 3 months). The major drawback to carnitine supplementation is the cost, which at doses of 1 to 3 g/d may range from $1 to 3/d.

V. COENZYME Q₁₀ (UBIQUINONE)

A. MECHANISMS OF ACTION

Coenzyme Q_{10} (ubiquinone) is a highly lipophilic compound that occupies a pivotal role in transfer of electrons produced from metabolism of foodstuffs to oxidative phosphorylation (electron transport chain), resulting in aerobic generation of adenosine triphosphate (ATP).[941] In addition to inhabiting inner mitochondrial membranes, coenzyme Q_{10} is also found in other cellular membranes, with functions as an antioxidant, membrane stabilizer, and redox activity being hypothesized.[941–943] Since coenzyme Q_{10} is essential for production of cellular energy under aerobic conditions, and since deficiencies of coenzyme Q_{10}, as shown by decreased plasma and tissue levels, are associated with decreased production of ATP and decreased organ function, the concentration of coenzyme Q_{10} as the single most essential metabolic component of ATP production is emphasized (for reviews, see[520–523,941,944–946]). Of even more interest for practical application is the finding that normal levels of coenzyme Q_{10} do not saturate the respiratory chain, and thus energy production, thereby leading to a working hypothesis that additional coenzyme Q_{10} would lead to increased cellular energy output, organ function, and physical performance.[947] This means that a rationale basis for coenzyme Q_{10} supplementation to increase aerobic exercise performance exists.

In both endurance-trained rats[524] and humans,[948,949] muscle coenzyme Q_{10} levels were increased over sedentary subjects, consistent with increased mitochondrial number and oxidative capacity induced by training.[549] However, plasma levels of coenzyme Q_{10} in trained cyclists[950] and endurance athletes[948,949] were significantly lower than sedentary controls. Increases in training intensity were associated with a further reduction in plasma coenzyme Q_{10} levels in trained cyclists.[950] An inverse correlation between plasma coenzyme Q_{10} levels and aerobic capacity was found for endurance runners.[951] Decreases in plasma, but not muscle, levels of coenzyme Q_{10} in trained athletes may be due to accelerated turnover or sequestration of coenzyme Q_{10} in muscles relative to metabolic demands.[948,951,952]

Rats supplemented with coenzyme Q_{10} and exercised for 90 min by downhill treadmill running exhibited prevention of elevated serum CPK and LDH enzymes seen in control groups.[525] Dietary supplementation of coenzyme Q_{10}, along with other antioxidant nutrients, was associated with decreases in lipid peroxidation in tissue slice assays.[526] These effects could be attributable to improvements in cellular energy production (delaying onset of exercise-induced muscle damage), membrane stabilization, or antioxidant activities, in support of hypothetical mechanisms of action for coenzyme Q_{10}.

B. HUMAN STUDIES

Supplementation with 100 mg/d of coenzyme Q_{10} for 6 weeks to endurance athletes increased both plasma and muscle coenzyme Q_{10} amounts by about 100%.[948] Thus, dietary coenzyme Q_{10} supplementation has been shown to enter muscle tissue and benefit biochemical parameters of importance to exercise performance, similar to dozens of other human studies.[520–523,941,944–946]

Data from the preceding studies indicated that coenzyme Q_{10} supplementation in athletes improves tissue saturation, a condition which may improve aerobic energy production, and perhaps performance. In six sedentary young men, one study found significant increases of 6 to 12% in submaximal and maximal exercise capacities 4 and 8 weeks after supplementation with 60 mg/d of coenzyme Q_{10}.[953] Myocardial contractility was also increased.

Twelve untrained male subjects were tested for blood levels of lactate, glucose, insulin, glycerol, nonesterified fatty acids (NEFA), and CPK before exercise, after 60 min of cycle ergometry at 50% VO_2max, followed by exhaustive work, and at 30 and 60 min post-exercise.[534] Coenzyme Q_{10} supplements (100 mg/d for 1 month) were given, and a followup exercise test with physiological measurements was performed. No significant changes were seen after coenzyme Q_{10} supplementation for all parameters, except for a significant decrease in NEFA levels during and immediately after exercise. The authors suggested that NEFA was utilized more efficiently as a fuel by exercising muscles.[534]

Nine middle-aged women complaining of easy fatigability demonstrated functional aerobic impairment without anemia or cardiovascular disease.[954] After 3 and 6 months of supplementation with 90 mg/d of coenzyme Q_{10}, treadmill tests to exhaustion were repeated. Subjects did not undergo physical training during the study period. At both 3 and 6 months, exercise time, peak oxygen intake (VO_2), and anaerobic threshold measurements were all significantly increased (improved). Peak heart rate and blood pressure were unaltered. Severity of symptoms improved for five of the nine subjects (three became normal). Thus, physical ability and aerobic exercise function was improved in sedentary subjects with decreased work ability.[954]

Twelve untrained male subjects were tested by graded cycle ergometer exercise to exhaustion after 60 min at 50% VO_2max before and after supplementation with 100 mg/d coenzyme Q_{10} for 30 d.[955] Blood glucose, insulin, lactate, CPK, glycerol, and NEFA levels were measured before exercise, at end of the aerobic phase of exercise, at exhaustion, and 30 and 60 min postexercise. The only significant difference between initial and post-supplement exercise tests was a substantial attenuation in the rise of NEFA during exercise.[955] Accelerated consumption of NEFA was postulated to explain the results, since a lipid-lowering effect of coenzyme Q_{10} in hyperlipidemic patients has been observed.[956]

Ten sedentary subjects and nine aerobically-trained volleyball players were studied in a double-blind, placebo-controlled crossover trial of supplementation with 100 mg/d of coenzyme Q_{10} or placebo for 30 d, with a 21 d withdrawal period.[957] Cycle ergometry with blood lactate determinations and cardiac performance measurements were performed at baseline and after each study period. After the coenzyme Q_{10} period, significant increases compared to baseline values were seen for: (1) total work capacity in both sedentary (1602 vs. 1242 W) and athletes (2737 vs. 2290) groups; (2) VO_2max in both sedentary (30 ± 4 vs. 25 ± 4 ml/min/kg) and athletic (40 ± 4 vs. 34 ± 4 ml/min/kg) groups; and (3) plasma coenzyme Q_{10} levels. No significant changes in maximal heart rate, peak lactate levels, or the product of blood pressure and heart rate were found. Except for a significant increase in VO_2max for the sedentary group (28 ± 4 vs. 25 ± 4 ml/min/kg), there were no significant changes from baseline values for any measurement after placebo administration. Thus, both sedentary subjects and anaerobic athletes showed improvement in aerobic performance after supplementation with coenzyme Q_{10}.

A double-blind crossover study administered 100 mg/d of coenzyme Q_{10} or placebo for 30 d to 18 endurance runners.[958] Plasma coenzyme Q_{10} levels at study onset were lower than a sedentary control group, but increased after coenzyme Q_{10} supplementation. After maximal exercise, average values of total oxygen consumption (VO_2, 25 ± 7 vs. 19 ± 7), lactic acid O_2 equivalent (2.9 ± 0.8 vs. 1.9 ± 0.9 L), total O_2 metabolized (25 ± 8 vs. 21 ± 7 L), VO_2max ($4 9 \pm 0.5$ vs. 3.8 ± 0.6 L/min), maximal work load (258 ± 41 vs. 247 ± 38 W), and total work (243 ± 61 vs. 217 ± 56 kJ) were significantly improved over the placebo period.[958] Levels of blood glucose, glycerol, and lactate were significantly increased 5 min post-exercise during the coenzyme Q_{10} period compared to the placebo period.

Twenty-two highly trained male endurance runners (150 to 170 km/week) were divided into two matched groups of 11 subjects each.[959] After initial tests, one group was given 100 mg/d of coenzyme Q_{10} for 40 d. Both groups performed similar training routines. Like other reports,[948-952] plasma levels of coenzyme Q_{10} were significantly lower than sedentary subjects (0.56 vs. 0.8-1.0 µg/ml). A graded treadmill run to exhaustion, preceded and followed by measurements of serum ammonia, uric acid, lactate, triglycerides, nonesterified fatty acids (NEFA), total cholesterol, CPK, and LDH was performed after 40 d. Both plasma (1.36 ± 0.40 vs. 0.58 ± 0.17 µg/ml) and platelet (62 ± 21 vs. 38 ± 18 pmol/mg prot) coenzyme Q_{10} levels increased significantly in the supplemented group, but not in the control group (0.49 ± 0.14 vs. 0.54 ± 0.20 µg/ml for serum). After exercise and during recovery (30 min post-exercise), the group supplemented with coenzyme Q_{10}, but not the control group, showed significantly lower levels of uric acid and triglycerides compared to initial test values. Compared to the control group, the supplemented group exhibited significantly lower levels of CPK (68 ± 31 vs. 216 ± 41 mU/ml), LDH (163 ± 55 vs. 318 ± 11 mU/ml), and ammonia/lactate ratios (1.4 ± 0.2 vs. 2.6 ± 0.8) after exercise.[959] Coenzyme Q_{10} administration appeared to enhance physiological parameters important to exercise performance that are consistent with postulated mechanisms of action.

Ten male professional basketball players were divided into two groups of five subjects each.[960] The supplemented group was given 100 mg/d of coenzyme Q_{10} for 40 d. Measurements of VO_2max and studies of heart function by echocardiographic and Doppler techniques were performed before and after the 40 d period. Athletes continued their normal training routines during the 40 d period. Plasma coenzyme Q_{10} levels doubled in the supplemented group (1.6 ± 0.5 vs. 0.85 ± 0.25 µg/ml), but were unchanged in the control group (0.87 ± 0.3 vs. 0.83 ± 0.1 µg/ml). VO_2max was significantly increased (18%) in the supplemented group (68 ± 2 vs. 56 ± 5 ml/min/kg), but not in the control group (55 ± 8 vs. 52 ± 8 ml/min/kg). After coenzyme Q_{10} administration, the supplemented group exhibited significant differences in the following cardiac performance parameters: (1) protodiastolic velocity; (2) ratio between protodiastolic and telediastolic velocity; (3) half pressure times; and (4) peak filling rates. Compared to the control group, the supplemented group exhibited significant differences in: (1) telediastolic velocity; (2) ratio between protodiastolic and telediastolic velocities; and (3) half pressure times. The control group showed no changes between measurements before and after 40 d. These results indicate improved aerobic capacity, cardiac efficiency, and performance of both systolic (contraction) and diastolic (relaxation) phases of heart functions after supplementation with coenzyme Q_{10} in athletes.[960]

Similar to studies with healthy people, administration of coenzyme Q_{10} to patients with cardiac ischemia and/or angina has repeatedly been associated with improvements in exercise tolerance and peak work capacity.[527–532,961–963]Thus, coenzyme Q_{10} supplementation should be considered for those initiating exercise programs as one component of physician-directed treatment for cardiovascular disease recovery.

C. SUMMARY AND GUIDELINES

Coenzyme Q_{10} supplementation has consistently shown improved physiological and physical parameters in both trained and untrained subjects, consistent with hypothetical mechanisms of action. Thus, coenzyme Q_{10} supplementation appears to be a viable option to improve aerobic performance. The long-term safety of coenzyme Q_{10} supplementation has been thoroughly documented in thousands of subjects.[520–523,941,944–946] Likewise, the ability of orally administered coenzyme Q_{10} to increase blood and tissue levels has also been extensively documented in both animals and humans.[520–523,941,944–946] Coenzyme Q_{10} is available at health food stores, mail order vitamin companies, and sporting goods stores. Attention to bioavailability is found for some products that offer coenzyme Q_{10} in oil, or emulsified. Thus, coenzyme Q_{10} is poised to be a nutritional ergogenic aid, providing further research studies confirm that performance in actual sports settings is improved.

Guidelines for use include any aerobic exercise, and patients with cardiovascular disease. Daily doses range from 60 to 200 mg/d. Similar to carnitine, this level of coenzyme Q_{10} supplementation would be expensive, ranging from $1 to 3/d.

VI. CREATINE

Creatine phosphate (phosphocreatine) serves as a reservoir of high-energy phosphate bonds in muscle and nerve tissues for maintenance of ATP levels during muscular activity that quickly deplete ATP.[52,535] Thus, increases in creatine phosphate levels should theoretically delay fatigue in repetitive, exhaustive, short-term exercise. Despite knowledge of creatine function since the early 1900s and availability of creatine commercially, only one report of creatine supplementation on human physical performance has been reported. In 1943, Beard published results of increased cycling times at constant workloads after creatine administration as cited by Keys.[198] However, no experimental details are available, so there exist no adequate studies of effects of creatine supplementation in humans.

Creatine is synthesized endogenously by the liver from arginine, glycine, and methyl donors.[535] Dietary creatine also influences muscle creatine pool size in man, with several studies reporting increases in muscle creatine after supplementation[536–539] or decreases after creatine-free diets.[536,540] Dietary creatine appears to be readily absorbed[536,537] and incorporated into tissues.[536,541] Since an average human contains approximately 115 g of creatine,[537] relatively large amounts of dietary creatine (1 g daily for several weeks or 10 g daily for 10 d) were required to produce noticeable increases in body creatine pool sizes. Thus, a hypothetical mechanism of action, proven bioavailability, and theoretically favorable change of creatine levels have been demonstrated after high doses of creatine supplementation. A need for determination of effects of creatine supplementation on exercise parameters remains. At present, no guidelines for use of creatine as an ergogenic aid are warranted.

VII. METHYL DONORS

Methyl donors comprise a group of compounds found in intermediary metabolism. Interactions with cobalamins and folate are implicit in methyl donor metabolism. Choline, betaine (trimethylglycine or TMG), dimethylglycine (DMG), sarcosine (N-methylglycine), methionine, and S-adenosyl methionine (SAM) are involved in transmethylation.[542] This process is essential for biosynthesis of several compounds important to muscle performance, primarily creatine and nucleic acids.[542]

A. LECITHIN (PHOSPHATIDYL CHOLINE)

Methyl donor supplementation to athletes has centered around two compounds: lecithin and DMG. Lecithin (soybean oil phospholipids containing 17 to 35% phosphatidyl choline) was the first inexpensive commercially available source of phosphatidyl choline. As such, it was believed to increase choline levels to aid creatine synthesis as well as to reinforce nerve and muscle cell membranes. Few reports on lecithin supplementation to athletes are found. An early German study administered 22 to 83 g of lecithin daily for several days to five subjects and reported beneficial effects on muscular power, endurance, and performance.[543] This study was refuted by Keys in 1943 on the basis of training effects and inadequate control.[198] Another study utilized a blind, crossover design with unsupplemented controls.[544] Grip strength was tested before and after 2 weeks of daily supplementation with 30 g of lecithin. No increases in strength were seen. Thus, lecithin has not been proved to be an effective ergogenic aid.

B. CHOLINE

Plasma choline levels have been demonstrated to decrease in runners after marathon races.[545] Decreases may theoretically impair acetylcholine release at neuromuscular junctions, leading to decreases in performance.[545] More work is needed to determine if this phenomenon is reproducible and significantly affects physical performance. Also, studies on effects of supplementation with lecithin and/or choline on athletes to replete the decreased choline levels have yet to be performed.

Even though both lecithin and choline supplementations have been shown to greatly increase blood choline levels,[546,547] few studies have been performed to correlate the increased blood levels with changes in transmethylation activity, creatine synthesis, or physical performance. Future research must take into account the low and variable phosphatidyl choline content of commercial lecithin[548] and the diarrhea and foul-smelling intestinal gas production from 20 g of choline base supplementation, although lower doses appeared safe.[549] Pure phosphatidyl choline and choline bitartrate forms may offer compatible supplements for future testing.

C. DIMETHYLGLYCINE (DMG) AND PANGAMIC ACID

DMG has enjoyed a checkered career. Initially, pangamic acid (vitamin B_{15}) was isolated from plant seeds, grain germs, and even mammalian tissues.[550] B_{15} was originally described as the dimethylaminoacetate of gluconic acid, and a commercially available form, calcium pangamate, was introduced and shown to increase utilization of oxygen by tissues in animals.[550] Russian research with calcium pangamate in rats reported increases of liver and muscle glycogen, muscle creatine phosphate, and muscle lipids, leading to decreased blood lactate levels after exercise.[551] Further Russian research on humans using 100 or 300 mg of calcium pangamate for 3 d showed a decrease in blood lactate after submaximal exercises (fencing, light track training, rowing, and cycle ergometry) when compared to a glucose placebo or no supplements.[552] Trends toward normalization of blood glucose and reduced/oxidized blood glutathione ratios were also noted for the pangamate users. The authors concluded pangamate increased oxygen utilization, but no statistical analysis was used. Because of these studies and uses of pangamate by Russian Olympic athletes in 1964 and 1968, as well as by popular American professional athletes, B_{15} or pangamate has achieved a cult status in the U.S., especially among runners.

Subsequent research has revealed considerable discrepancies in the composition of the compound characterized by Krebs.[553] Frequently, calcium gluconate and DMG were mixed together and labeled as a pangamate. N,N-diisopropylamine dichloroacetate, glucono-di-(N-diisopropylamino) acetate, and glycine have also been marketed as vitamin B_{15} or pangamate.[553,554] Furthermore, in an unsuccessful effort to discourage indiscriminate use[555] the FDA has proclaimed B_{15} to be a food additive of unknown composition, and thus it cannot be sold in pure form (to meet safety regulations). For these reasons, analysis of study results must consider the chemical identity of the "pangamate" or "B_{15}" used.

Only one published study has reported beneficial ergogenic effects after "pangamic acid" supplementation.[556] Twelve track athletes were divided into two groups, one of which received 5 mg of pangamic acid (uncharacterized) for 7 d. The other group received a placebo. A treadmill run to exhaustion was measured before and after the supplementation period. Subjects receiving pangamic acid showed an average increase in time to exhaustion of 24% and increases in VO_2max of 28%. The placebo group showed increases of 1% and 3% respectively. Since the study was reported in an abstract, no other details were available.

Other studies utilizing DMG (with or without calcium gluconate) reported significant increases in human performance. One study found increased work tolerance and decreased blood lactate levels after DMG administration.[557] An unpublished dissertation cited by Gray and Titlow[555] claimed 30% lower lactate levels following exercise than a placebo group after 4 weeks of DMG supplementation. Dosage was not reported. Animal studies employing racing greyhounds[558] or racing horses[559] found improvements in performance times and blood lactate levels, respectively, after oral DMG dosing. One study on rats found no enhancement of performance or liver transmethylation activities after DMG injections.[560]

A randomized, blind crossover study administered six tablets of an equimolar mixture of calcium gluconate (61.5% by weight) and DMG (38.5% by weight) for a presumed daily dose of 115.5 mg of DMG for 2 weeks.[561,562] No effects of DMG consumption were seen for VO_2, oxygen debt, oxygen deficit, heart rate, blood lactate, or R values during and after cycle ergometry at 76% VO_2max. Using the same dosage form, amount, and length of administration as the previous study, another report found no effects of DMG on VO_2max, anaerobic threshold, or 15-min run times.[563] Eighteen male subjects were used in a counterbalanced design with control, placebo, and DMG groups. Likewise, another double-blind experiment found no significant changes in heart rate, treadmill run times to exhaustion, blood glucose levels, or blood lactate levels when compared to the placebo group and the pretreatment period for 16 track athletes ingesting 115.5 mg/d of DMG for 21 d.[564] Twenty active males were given 200 mg/d of DMG or a placebo for 21 d, followed by a period of time to allow for any residual effects to subside, then a crossover period.[565] No effect of DMG on heart rate, VO_2max, treadmill, or anaerobic threshold was seen. A graded maximal exercise treadmill test was used. One double-blind, crossover, counter-balanced study on effects of acute DMG supplementation (135 mg immediately prior to a treadmill run) found no effects on performance or physiological responses from 16 trained runners.[566] Thus, results from five well-controlled studies did not find beneficial ergogenic effects from DMG (the active component of B_{15} or pangamic acid preparations) in submaximal or maximal exercises. Whether a larger dose of DMG or a longer supplementation period would change performance parameters has not been measured.

1. DMG Safety

It was formerly believed that a reason to avoid large oral doses of DMG existed. DMG had been shown to be converted to nitrososarcosine, a weak carcinogen, in mouse stomachs.[567] Nitrite presence greatly increased the amount of nitrososarcosine formed. Nitrites are present in human saliva and many preserved meat products. Another form of commercial pangamic acid, DIPA-dichloroacetate, was shown to be mutagenic by the Ames test.[568] It appears that many dietary tertiary amines are being considered as nitrosatable compounds capable of causing cancer in humans. However, recent work has cast doubt on the risk of carcinogen formation from DMG.[569,570] First, the risk of formation of nitroso compounds from dietary levels of DMG and similar compounds is very low (less than 1 fmol of nitrosated DMG products), even if supplemental amounts (100 mg/d) are factored.[569] Second, extensive repeat experiments with more rigorous procedural controls have not found mutagenic activity from DMG reacted with nitrite.[570]

2. Summary and Guidelines

In summary, DMG has not shown consistent ergogenic effects in several well-controlled studies. However, dose-response and length of administration effects on exercise performance have yet to be determined.

Studies of effects of methyl donors on exercise performance have centered on only two of many possible compounds. One (lecithin) has not been studied recently in forms known to produce increases in tissue choline and acetylcholine levels. Uses of compounds such as methionine, S-adenosyl methionine, choline bitartrate, betaine, or choline biosynthetic precursors, such as the various folate forms, have not been adequately examined in regard to exercise performance. Thus, guidelines for use of phosphatidyl choline, choline, or DMG as ergogenic aids would be premature at this time.

VIII. NUCLEIC ACIDS (INOSINE AND ADENINE)

A. INOSINE

Inosine is both a precursor and a breakdown product of adenosine.[571] Increases of inosine in cells are thought to force additional synthesis of adenosine (and ultimately ATP) by providing precursors and inhibiting catabolism of adenine nucleotides. Inosine may also contribute to nucleotide pools for DNA, RNA, and protein synthesis. Also, inosine is thought to improve oxygen utilization because of its effects on erythrocyte metabolism.[572] Inosine is used *in vitro* to maintain viability of stored erythrocytes.[573] In French clinical trials, parenteral inosine has shown benefit in therapy for cardiac insufficiency, angina, digitalis toxicity, extrasystoles, and senility in older patients.[574,575] These results were attributed to inotropic hormone-like effects rather than enhancement of cellular ATP levels.[576]

Currently, inosine is widely touted by several companies as an effective energy booster, based on testimonials and rumors of use by Russian and Eastern Bloc athletes. One report on inosine administration was found in a nonpeer-reviewed popular magazine.[577] Four trained weightlifters were given either a placebo or 3 g/d of inosine for 6 weeks in a double-blind, matched pairs, crossover study. Changes in one-, five-, and eight-repetition maxima (RM) for four exercises were measured, although only one RM was reported. Average strength gains seemed to be improved after inosine dosing. However, no statistical analysis was presented, and the investigator commented that constant use of inosine tended to exhaust athletes.

In humans, excess inosine is not converted to adenine nucleotides, but is metabolized by the enzyme xanthine oxidase, a potent generator of superoxide radicals,[578] to uric acid.[579,580] In humans, liver and small intestines contain large amounts of xanthine oxidase.[581] Importantly, xanthine dehydrogenase in muscle tissue is converted to active xanthine oxidase by ischemia and exercise,[350,581,582] increasing the formation of free radicals in muscle tissue to a greater extent than explained by resting levels of muscle xanthine oxidase. This mechanism is now thought to be a major generator of exercise-induced free radicals and lipid peroxidation. In fact, plasma inosine, hypoxanthine, and uric acid levels are used as markers for ischemia and anaerobic stress.[583–586] Exacerbation of gout by excess purines is also possible after administration of inosine.[223,587] Furthermore, oral administration of purine nucleotides (e.g., inosine or adenosine) to rodents reveals substantial degradation by the intestinal mucosa,[588] rendering oral supplementation of inosine to have at best, dubious, and at worst, hazardous value to humans.

B. ADENINE

Adenine, however, is well absorbed from the diet and incorporated into nucleotides *in vivo*.[589] Adenine is also commonly used to preserve stored erythrocytes,[590] and was named vitamin B_4 until its nonessentiality was proven.[553] Sublingual and parenteral administration of adenosine and adenosine phosphates by German clinicians have been reported to lower serum cholesterol,[591] improve angina and atherosclerotic senility,[591] and prevent recurrence of secondary myocardial infarcts.[592] However, no reports of oral adenine or adenosine supplementation on athletic performance have been found. In addition, adenine supplementation may lead to renal tubular damage caused by formation of the insoluble metabolite 2,8-dihydroxyadenine, as has been seen in dogs.[593] In conclusion, the mechanism of action of purine supplements as ergogenic aids may deserve further study in animals, but potential toxicities may render human testing and use hazardous. At this time, no guidelines for use of inosine or other nucleotides as ergogenic aids are apparent.

Chapter 5

MICRONUTRIENT SUPPLEMENTATION AND ERGOGENESIS — MINERALS

I. INTRODUCTION

This section will describe research results of mineral supplementation on exercise performance, excluding the electrolytes sodium, potassium, and chloride, which have been discussed elsewhere previously.

The only nonelectrolyte minerals studied in any detail are calcium, magnesium, zinc, iron, selenium, chromium and phosphorus (as phosphate). Other minerals such as cobalt, copper, iodine, manganese, vanadium, molybdenum, lithium, rubidium, cesium, germanium, tin, etc. have not been studied specifically as ergogenic aids in humans. The only trace minerals at this time with a theoretical rationale for use are zinc (to correct possible deficiencies), rubidium and cesium (to change intracellular pH), chromium (to affect carbohydrate and amino acid metabolism via effects on insulin), selenium (as an antioxidant), and vanadium (for insulin receptor effects).

II. CALCIUM

One early report suggested that daily ingestion of calcium gluconate aids recovery from exercise, but no details are available.[594] A recent study examined the effect of hypertonic calcium (1 to 1.45 l of a 1.5% solution of calcium gluconate) on plasma volume during rest, during exercise at 40 to 47% VO_2max, and during recovery in both cold and hot climates.[595] Prevention of the normal hypervolemic response of plasma after fluid ingestion was seen at rest and during exercise in heat (39.4°C). This phenomenon attenuates temperature elevations during exercise.[596]

Calcium supplements have also been used to prevent and treat osteoporosis in females, especially older women. Osteoporosis causes acute problems in 6.3 million people in the U.S.,[597] and leads to 1.3 million fractures yearly.[598] It is believed that chronic intake of insufficient amounts of calcium, excessive amounts of phosphorus, lack of exercise, aging, and postmenopausal loss of estrogen contribute to formation of osteoporosis.[597,598] Two-thirds of U.S. women between the ages of 18 to 30 (when peak bone mass is attained) consume less than the RDA for calcium (1000 mg/d).[597] Incidence of prolonged amenorrhea secondary to exercise in female athletes ranges from 7 to 43%, leading to further losses of bone mass in thinner subjects.[599,600] For these reasons, dietary changes to increase calcium content are necessary for most postpubertal females. Calcium supplementation may be considered in order to achieve a consistent intake. Both exercise[601–604] and calcium supplements[597,598,602,605] have been shown to prevent loss of bone mineral in nonosteoporotic, middle-aged (30 to 60 years old) and elderly women (over 60 years old), although when calcium supplements (750 mg/d) and exercise were combined, no additive effect was seen in elderly women.[602] Calcium supplements alone have generally not improved bone mass in severely osteoporotic elderly patients, possibly due to absorption difficulties.[606]

Muscle cramps may be partly caused by calcium losses from the sarcoplasmic reticulum of muscle tissue, leading to altered neuromuscular function and impaired muscle glycogen breakdown.[607] Although calcium is lost in sweat,[607] it appears that acclimatization and small (100 to 150mg) increases in dietary calcium can decrease calcium losses to the point of prevention of calcium-deficient muscle cramps.[607]

Interestingly, calcium supplementation has been used in many ergogenic studies as a placebo for control groups. Many of the studies analyzing the effects of sodium bicarbonate or ammonium chloride on exercise utilized calcium carbonate ($CaCO_3$) as a placebo.[361-363,365,367,382,383,404,608] Since dietary calcium absorption in normal persons ranges from 30 to 60%,[609] perhaps the prevention of plasma volume increase caused greater than usual changes in blood parameters such as glucose or lactate. The effect of calcium on the outcome of such studies remains to be elucidated.

Calcium gluconate is also a component of "pangamic acid" supplements tested as ergogenic acids.[552,561-564] However, doses of supplemental calcium would not exceed 20 mg, a very small dose. The absence of increases in performance seen by four studies using calcium gluconate and DMG also suggests that such low amounts of calcium do not improve performance.[561-564] Thus, research on the effects of calcium supplementation are few and generally do not indicate a need for or benefit from calcium supplementation, except for thin, amenorrheic female athletes.

In cases were bone mass is reduced, or in thin, amenorrheic women, guidelines for calcium supplementation are daily doses of 500 to 1000 mg of calcium, preferably from calcium citrate, calcium citrate/malate, calcium gluconate, or calcium lactate. Increases of dietary calcium from dairy products (preferably low-fat or non-fat dairy products) and green leafy vegetables are also advised.

III. MAGNESIUM

Magnesium losses in sweat can become significant if sweating is profuse.[607,610] One case report described the successful cessation of carpopedal spasms in a female tennis player with hypomagnesemia after daily supplementation with 500 mg of magnesium gluconate (29 mg of elemental magnesium).[610] Endurance athletes are at high risk for developing magnesium deficiencies, with suspected detriments to performance.[611] In fact, only one report has studied magnesium supplementation to athletes, and enhanced physical capacity was found.[612] Given the importance of magnesium for cellular functions, and probable widespread marginal intakes,[611] it seems prudent to initiate research on the role of magnesium in exercise.

Guidelines for magnesium supplementation (when known to be depleted) are 100 to 250 mg/d of magnesium from magnesium lactate, magnesium gluconate, magnesium glycinate, magnesium taurate, or magnesium chloride.

IV. IRON

The importance of iron for oxygen transport via hemoglobin and endurance exercise has been well documented.[647] Female athletes in particular frequently exhibit subnormal levels of hemoglobin and "sports anemia".[607,613] Iron supplementation to anemic persons (including athletes) has improved hemoglobin concentration, red blood cell count, hematocrit, VO_2max, maximal work times, heart rate responses, and performance times.[614-621] Iron supplementation to nonanemic, iron-deficient athletes has generally resulted in increases of hemoglobin, serum iron, or tissue stores.[622-626] Decreases in lactate levels after exercise have been attributed to iron supplementation, but no changes in VO_2max or time to exhaustion have been seen.[623,625-629] One study found improvements in exercise performance from nonanemic, iron-deficient athletes after iron therapy.[630]

Iron supplements to athletes with normal iron status have been shown in a few studies to improve iron status.[607,623,631] Other studies have not found changes in iron status.[615,632-637] In the only study that examined performance after iron supplementation, no changes in VO_2max were found, although the subjects were sedentary.[615]

In summary, iron supplementation appears beneficial to iron-deficient athletes, especially if anemia is involved. Effects of iron supplements on the performance of athletes with normal iron status are yet to be reported. Risk factors that need to be examined to determine whether sports anemia is present include (1) dietary analysis of protein, iron, copper, vitamin C, vitamin B_{12}, and folate intakes; (2) iron loss rates (such as menstruation or hemolysis due to excessive running); (3) iron status (determined by a physician requesting and analyzing clinical laboratory tests); and (4) very intense training, especially the beginning of a program.[607] More research is needed to determine fully the effects of iron supplementation. Research is justified, since iron deficiency is not uncommon in the general population as well as in athletes.[607]

Guidelines for iron supplementation to anemic and/or iron-deficient, nonanemic individuals are 25 to 75 mg/d, preferably as ferrous fumarate, ferrous lactate, ferrous bis-glycinate, or iron-dextran complexes to avoid common side effects of nausea, constipation, and gastritis from ferrous sulfate preparations.

V. PHOSPHATES

Use of phosphates to influence physical performance started with Embden (of the Embden-Meyerhof pathway) during the First World War. German soldiers in the field (including whole battalions) were given foods and drink rich in phosphorus as well as supplements of sodium acid phosphate.[638] Early

German research proclaimed that phosphates reduced fatigue of athletes and workers.[639–647] Early Russian and European work also reported that 1 to 3 g of sodium acid phosphate, taken 1 h before exercise but not 5 to 10 g taken 9 to 10 h before exercise, improved psychomotor performance, elevated heart rate, elevated skin temperatures, reduced sweat production, and prevented the increase due to fatigue in muscular stimulation time as recorded by Moss's ergograph.[648–658] Unfortunately, most of these studies have been criticized for lack of data, lack of controls, or subjective measurements of fatigue or performance.[198] Keller and Kraut reported results of Rogoskin on supplementation with 2 g of sodium dihydrogen phosphate 1 h prior to exercise on 190 athletes engaged in running, rowing, and swimming.[659] All athletes on phosphates reported improvements, whereas less than half of unsupplemented athletes showed improvements. These results were subject to training and placebo effects, and no statistical analysis was presented.

A recent study examined effects of phosphate loading on physiological parameters.[660] Ten trained, male distance runners were given 1 g of neutral-buffered phosphate four times daily or a crossover placebo consisting of 0.1 g sodium citrate four times daily in a double-blind manner for 3 d before exercise. An intermittent graded, treadmill run to exhaustion was used to measure VO_2max. Sequence of administration was a control period, followed by three experimental periods (two phosphate, one placebo), and a final control period, with each period being separated by 1 week. A significant increase in pre-exercise serum phosphate and erythrocyte 2,3-diphosphoglycerate (2,3-DPG) was found after oral phosphate loading. Increases in mid-exercise blood lactate were decreased during phosphate loading trials. VO_2max was also significantly increased. It also appeared that elevation of 2,3-DPG remained for over 1 week after phosphate supplementation, as indicated by comparison of results when the placebo period came prior to or after phosphate periods. Performance times were not recorded, although subjects were reported to run from one to three grades more during all phosphate periods and some placebo periods. This study shows that short-term phosphate loading appears to improve aerobic capacity by altering 2,3-DPG levels to a favorable degree (similar to those induced by changes in altitude or exercise training[659]).

Another recent study examined the effects of phosphate loading on leg power and high-intensity treadmill runs on 11 graduate physical education majors.[661] Both acute and chronic effects of phosphate were measured. Acute effects were measured 1 h after ingestion of 1.24 g of sodium and potassium phosphate (Stim-O-Stam), while chronic administration consisted of 3.73 g/d for 6 d prior to testing. Supplements and placebos (white flour) were administered in a double-blind complete cross-over manner. Exhaustive treadmill running times were not affected by either acute or chronic phosphate loading. Time for a second treadmill run to exhaustion, started 15 min after the end of the first run, was also not affected by phosphates. Leg power measured by an isokinetic dynamometer showed no changes. Oxygen consumption (VO^2) during the treadmill runs was also not affected by phosphate administration.

Thus, no beneficial effects of phosphates were seen. Physiological parameters, such as blood lactate or erythrocyte 2,3-DPG, were not measured.

Discrepancies between results of the last two studies may relate to differences in the training status of the subjects, the types of exercise performed, and the doses of phosphate administered. Further research on large amounts of phosphate salts as an ergogenic aid is necessary before further broad conclusions can be drawn. The early German and Russian research indicates that long-term administration of phosphate is well tolerated and makes phosphate loading an attractive candidate for further research as an ergogenic aid. Advances in the use of NMR in following intracellular or tissue phosphate moieties promise to provide new insights into phosphate metabolism, important for a better understanding of ergogenic properties for phosphates.[662]

At this time, no definitive guidelines for phosphate supplementation as an ergogenic aid are presented.

VI. ZINC

Even though there is growing concern that zinc nutriture may not be ideal in many athletes,[663] insufficient data has accumulated to determine whether zinc supplementation would have potential ergogenic effects.

VII. SELENIUM

The primary role of selenium is to provide activity for glutathione peroxidase (GPx), a major cellular antioxidant.[664] Deficiencies of selenium are associated with Keshan disease (cardiomyopathy), Kashin-Beck disease (osteoarthritis), cardiomyopathies, and muscle weakness,[664] signifying that selenium deficiencies may decrease exercise performance, but these situations may not be applicable to healthy athletes. As part of the antioxidant defense system, selenium may play a role in prevention of fatigue or may aid recovery from exhaustive exercise (see section on antioxidants).

Supplemental selenium (0.15 ppm in diet for 4 weeks) to race horses prevented the post-exercise rise in serum of muscle enzymes and of malondialdehyde (MDA) levels (a measure of free radical damage).[665] The same investigators did not find differences in swimming times or MDA levels of rats fed various levels of selenium.[666] An injection of selenium (25 mg) plus vitamin E (55 mg) to racehorses, followed by vigorous exercise, resulted in lower plasma lipid peroxide levels.[667]

A report from the Sports Polyclinic in Romania employed 33 elite swimmers in a crossover study involving selenium supplementation.[668] After supplementation with 150 mcg selenium (as selenite) for 2 weeks, post-exercise levels of serum lipid peroxides were significantly reduced, and post-exercise decreases in serum nonproteic sulfhydryls (glutathione) were spared. These results illustrate that selenium supplementation at levels within the recommended daily amounts can benefit antioxidant status of athletes. The observed changes may be of significance to athletes, and argue for increased research attention for selenium as an ergogenic, or protective, aid.

Other than as a component of antioxidant vitamin mixtures (see section on antioxidants), guidelines for selenium supplementation as an ergogenic aid are premature.

VIII. CHROMIUM

The essential qualities of chromium relate to its function as the Glucose Tolerance Factor (GTF) and its involvement with insulin metabolism.[669] Thus, chromium is required for efficient handling of carbohydrate, fats, and amino acids. Chromium deficiencies may be widespread due to low dietary intakes,[670] and initial research suggests that exercise may increase excretion of chromium.[671-673] These findings put athletes at risk for developing chromium deficiencies, with resulting insulin intolerance.

Evans administered 200 mcg of trivalent chromium (as chromium picolinate) daily in two separate studies on collegiate weightlifters.[674] The first study found significant increases in lean body mass for the supplemented group, compared to a placebo group (+2.2 vs. +0.4 kg), and less body fat percentage (0.0 vs. +1.1%) after 40 d. Ten total subjects attending a weight-lifting class twice weekly served as subjects. The second study divided 31 football players in a supervised weightlifting program for 6 weeks into two groups. The supplemented group received 200 mcg of chromium (as picolinate) daily, and compared to the placebo group, showed larger gains in lean body mass (2.6 vs. 1.8 kg) and greater decreases in body fat percentage (3.6 vs. 1.2%).[674] Another study by Hasten et al. gave 200 mcg/d of chromium (as picolinate) to 37 males and 22 females in a 12 week weightlifting program.[675] Supplemented females showed a greater increase in lean body mass than did control group females. No significant differences between the male groups were found.

Although these studies had some flaws,[675] they suggest that chromium may have desirable effects for weightlifters. However, at this time, whether a true ergogenic effect of chromium or simply repletion of marginally deficient states was observed has not been differentiated. Because of the need for safe alternatives for anabolic steroid abuse, safety of chromium supplements, benefits seen in preliminary studies, an attractive mechanism of action, potential losses of chromium due to exercise and sweating, and possible widespread dietary deficiencies or imbalances of chromium for the entire U.S. population, further attention should be focused on chromium as a potential ergogenic aid for weightlifters. The chromium status of endurance athletes, especially those consuming a diet high in refined carbohydrates, should also be examined.

Presently, no guidelines for chromium supplementation as an ergogenic aid are substantiated.

Chapter 6

MICRONUTRIENT SUPPLEMENTATION AND ERGOGENESIS — AMINO ACIDS

I. INTRODUCTION

Although several dozen individual, purified amino acids have been commercially available for many years and have been used extensively by clinicians, few have been applied to enhance athletic performance, and fewer still have been tested objectively for effects on physiological parameters important to exercise metabolism. This section will not investigate changes in amino acid metabolism after exercise; rather, reports on various single amino acids that describe effects on physical performance or metabolic processes of interest to exercise will be presented.

II. ARGININE

A. SOMATOTROPIN RELEASE

Arginine is known to influence several metabolic parameters important to exercise. First, i.v. infusion of arginine releases significant amounts of the anabolic hormones somatotropin (growth hormone)[676-684] and prolactin.[685-687] Consistency of this effect has led to the arginine infusion test as a clinical procedure to determine growth hormone status of humans.[688,689] Doses used to elicit a release of growth hormone ranged from 15 to 30 g, leading to a four- to sixfold increase in plasma arginine levels. Whether a similar blood level can be obtained after p.o. arginine loading has not been well studied. Clinical observations have revealed that 6 g of oral arginine increases plasma levels by 100% with no release of growth hormone.[690] Regardless of these results, use of p.o. arginine to increase growth hormone levels has become popular, propagated by anecdotal comments in a popular book.[691]

Evidence that oral arginine administration can stimulate somatotropin secretion is found in European research with arginine and arginine aspartate. Mathieni et al. found that after 5 d of oral arginine supplementation (5 g/d) to 12 subjects, the somatotropin response to intravenous arginine was blunted, but the response to intravenous insulin was enhanced.[692] In addition, low dose, intravenous arginine infusion studies found that a rise of 52% in serum arginine was sufficient to account for a significant rise in serum somatotropin levels.[692] Increases in sleep-related somatotropin and prolactin secretion were observed after chronic (7 d) administration of oral arginine aspartate (250 mg/kg/d) to five normal subjects.[693] No effects were seen at oral doses of 100 mg/kg/d. A large, single oral dose of arginine aspartate (37.5 g) caused a small but significant release of serum somatotropin in 12 normal adults.[694] Thus, there is evidence that acute or chronic administration of arginine (as the dipeptide arginine aspartate) can either stimulate release of somatotropin or enhance ability of other stimuli to release somatotropin.

Arginine pyroglutamate (L-arginine-2-pyrrolidone-5-carboxylate) was combined with L-lysine hydrochloride (1200 mg of each) and administered orally to 15 healthy male volunteers aged 15 to 20 years.[695] Biologically active growth hormone was greatly elevated in plasma from 30 to 120 min after the p.o. dose (two to eight times baseline value). Plasma somatomedin A levels were trebled at 8 h after administration. Plasma insulin levels were doubled at 30 min after oral dosing of the mixture. Administration of arginine pyroglutamate or lysine by themselves did not result in a significant increase of growth hormone over baseline levels. Nevertheless, although use of oral arginine supplementation to release somatotropin is possible, there is still much controversy over whether increased somatotropin levels (if indeed, levels are continually released) are of benefit to athletes.[10]

B. CREATINE SYNTHESIS

Second, arginine is a precursor for creatine synthesis.[542] Similar to glycine, arginine supplementation (equimolar amounts of glycine and arginine at 4 g of nitrogen daily) increased the rate of synthesis of creatine.[536] The increased synthetic rate was calculated to achieve a small increase in body creatine stores. Whether this increase in creatine would be sufficient to influence performance is unknown.

C. AMMONIA DETOXIFICATION

Third, arginine is an intermediate in the urea cycle.[686] The urea cycle converts ammonia (toxic to the body) into urea, a relatively harmless waste product. Ammonia is produced during exercise and may be one major factor in determination of fatigue.[697-699] Deamination of AMP by muscle cells is thought to be the primary source of ammonia during exercise.[698,699] This ammonia rapidly diffuses to the bloodstream, where elevated levels interfere with γ-aminobutyric acid (GABA) actions in brain, in synaptic neurophysiological control, and in loss of ATP used to detoxify the excess ammonia.[699] Ammonia production is greater during intense exercise (greater than 40 to 70% VO$_2$max); it increases use of fast-twitch muscle fibers and may be a more accurate measure of exercise intensity or muscle fiber type composition than blood lactate levels.[699] Ammonia formation may also provide a marker for free-radical formation during exercise (from actions of xanthine oxidase on inosine metabolites).[699]

Arginine supplementation to reduce ammonia toxicity has been demonstrated in animal models, where toxic doses of ammonia were produced by ammonium salts or excessive amino acid intake.[700-711] Human subjects who were administered i.v. amino acids to induce blood ammonia increases or patients with elevated ammonia levels also showed decreases in ammonia levels after 1 to 4 g of i.v. arginine.[697,709,712] Administration of arginine to athletes with determination of plasma ammonia levels after exercise has not been performed. Clinical results, availability, and safety of p.o. arginine loading suggest a need for further testing on reduction of exercise-induced ammonia levels during high-intensity exercises.

D. HUMAN EXERCISE

Eighteen untrained adult males initiated a 5 week resistance training program (three workouts per week).[713] Ten subjects received 1 g each of arginine and ornithine split into two daily doses, while eight subjects received a placebo. After 5 weeks, body fat decreased significantly more in the supplemented group (–0.85 vs. –0.20%), body mass decreased significantly more in the supplemented group (–1.3 vs. –0.81 kg), but composite muscle girth changes were equivalent. Results suggested that oral arginine/ornithine supplementation reduced body fat and mass to a greater degree when combined with a resistance training program for untrained, sedentary adult males.

E. SUMMARY AND GUIDELINES

Thus, several mechanisms with supportive evidence in humans suggest that p.o. loading of arginine may benefit performance of athletes, particularly weightlifters. Both acute (to reduce ammonia levels and possibly affect growth hormone levels) and chronic (to influence muscle mass and creatine levels) modes of administration should be considered in future studies.

At this time, guidelines for use of arginine supplements as an ergogenic aid for weightlifters are only speculative. Chronic, high-dose supplementation (2 to 10 g/d) is suggested by the literature as possibly effective for enhanced reduction of body fat during resistance training. Further studies at these dose levels in trained individuals are indicated before guidelines on arginine supplementation can be regarded as indicative.

III. ASPARTIC ACID

Effects of aspartate salts on human performance have been reviewed in a previous section of this book. This section will be concerned with aspartic acid itself. Animal studies have shown that aspartic acid administration can reduce ammonia blood levels after exercise.[463,714] Likewise, elevated ammonia levels have been reduced or prevented in animals after aspartic acid administration (singly or in combination with other amino acids.)[715–717] Corresponding doses (over 5 g) in humans have not been associated with any toxicity.[718] No studies have yet to investigate the relationship of aspartic acid intake and ammonia production after exercise in humans undergoing intense exercise.

The section on arginine included studies on effects of arginine aspartate, which are hypothesized to be mainly due to the arginine moiety.

No guidelines for use of aspartic acid as an ergogenic aid for humans are apparent.

IV. BRANCHED-CHAIN AMINO ACIDS (BCAAS)

Leucine, isoleucine, and valine make up the indispensable branched-chain amino acids (BCAA). Much clinical use has documented the beneficial effects (increase in nitrogen retention) of BCAA in various conditions, especially in hepatic coma, postsurgical trauma, starvation, and parenteral nutrition.[719-722]

Athletes showed decreased serum levels of leucine and isoleucine.[723] Intravenous administration of leucine (20 to 30 g) showed a similar release of growth hormone as did arginine.[677,684] Insulin is also released by i.v. leucine.[724] Isoleucine and valine showed less release of growth hormone than leucine.[677] However, p.o. supplementation of BCAA with measurement of resultant serum growth hormone levels in humans has not been reported.

Leucine can serve as an energy substrate in muscle,[719-721] and BCAA are selectively taken up by peripheral tissues (muscles).[725] Thus, supplementation with BCAA would appear to be desirable for athletes, especially both as an energy source and as a potential anabolic (nitrogen-sparing) agent. No studies using BCAA to enhance muscle growth in human athletes have been reported. Therefore, no substantiated guidelines for BCAA oral supplementation to exercising humans exist.

V. GLUTAMATE

Muscle tissue is able to reduce intracellular ammonia levels by addition of the ammonia to glutamate to form glutamine.[698,699] This reaction is catalyzed by the enzyme glutamine synthetase and ATP.[698,699] Training induces higher rates of glutamine synthetase activity.[698,699]

Glutamate supplementation, both p.o. and i.v. as monosodium glutamate (MSG), has been shown to reduce plasma ammonia levels in humans with hepatic failure.[707,726-728] One report administered 9 g of MSG i.v. to six healthy, untrained men followed by exercise to exhaustion on a cycle ergometer.[729] The level of blood ammonia produced was halved with glutamate, compared to saline infusion. Lactate, pyruvate, uric acid, glucose, and urea values were not changed significantly by glutamate infusion. No performance measurements were made, but since MSG infusion at the rate of 200 mg/min produced nausea in most subjects, subjective tolerance of exercise was less. The authors concluded that MSG could reduce ammonia levels produced by exercise, but practical use appears ill advised.

MSG has been shown to be more toxic than glutamic acid in subjects with "Chinese Restaurant Syndrome".[730] Nausea and vomiting have been known to occur when serum glutamic acid levels are increased 20-fold.[730] Perhaps p.o. administration of glutamic acid, but not MSG, would alleviate nausea. These studies have not yet been performed in conjunction with physical performance.

Use of the dipeptide, arginine glutamate, has been suggested as preventing electrolyte imbalance in patients where either arginine hydrochloride or MSG would otherwise be administered.[697] Preliminary clinical experience showed equivalent effectiveness of arginine or glutamate.[697] However, at this time there are no guidelines for use of glutamates as an ergogenic aid.

VI. GLYCINE

Glycine (aminoacetic acid or Glycocoll) was studied in detail during the 1930s and 1940s, but very little since then. Early interest in glycine as an ergogenic aid was stimulated by clinical trials of glycine on muscular dystrophy and myasthenia gravis patients.[731] Both illnesses exhibit muscle weakness and/or creatine loss from muscle tissue. Thus, the creatine precursor glycine was given to these patients with modest success.[732-745] When glycine was administered to normal persons, reductions in fatigue were reported, but this could be accounted for by psychological effects.[737,746-748]

A. HUMAN EXERCISE

Glycine administration to athletes or exercising subjects has produced ambiguous results. Significant increases in muscle strength as measured by the Rogers Strength Index after ingestion of 6 g of glycine daily for 10 weeks was noted in 1941.[749] Endurance (ratio of 220 to 60 yd run times) was not affected. A placebo group was employed. Grip strengths may not have been accurate due to positioning of the body on the dynamometer used. Strength measurements included chin pull-ups, push-ups, back lift, and leg lift. Cycle ergometry workloads after ingestion of 5 to 12 g daily of glycine showed increases of 22% for women and 32% for men.[745] In addition, constant work rates were maintained longer after glycine, glycine plus urea, or glycine plus urea plus phosphate. However, training effects were not controlled.

Another report found no increases in strength of the extensor digitorum communis (forearm) muscles of two subjects consuming 15 g of glycine for 30 d.[750] Six or twelve grams of glycine daily for 10 weeks did not improve grip strength of eight men, although urine creatine levels were increased.[751] Thirty-three football players were given a placebo or 5 g of glycine daily (except Sundays or holidays when 4.5 g were consumed) for 21 d in a double-blind crossover manner.[752] No differences in work output at a rate of 144 W/s from a cycle ergometer were noticed.

No further studies were reported until 1964 when 1.5 g of glycine or glycine plus 150 mg niacin were given to 86 subjects at either 2 h, 1 h, 4 min or immediately before exercise.[753] No effects on cycle ergometry or elbow flexion ergometry were seen.

Glycine as contained in gelatin protein has also been studied as an ergogenic aid. Results are described in the section on gelatin (Chapter 8, Section IV) in this book. No recent experiments on the ergogenic effects of glycine have been presented, nor have any measurements of muscle creatine synthesis or concentrations simultaneous with physical performance measurements been reported.

B. OTHER PROPERTIES

Typical or usual dietary consumption of glycine, a dispensable amino acid, is 3 to 5 g,[754] while 13 to 17 g daily are synthesized by the body.[755] Obviously, in order to influence body handling of glycine, large amounts (over several grams at once) must be taken; 30 g of p.o. glycine elevate serum glycine levels fourfold and also increase growth hormone levels to ten times over baseline 2 h after ingestion.[754] This amount of glycine was well tolerated. Oral administration of 6.75 g glycine to 19 subjects increased growth hormone significantly for 3 h, peaking at 3 to 4 times baseline at 2 h.[756] Likewise, i.v. infusion of 4, 8, or 12 g of glycine led to increases in serum growth hormone.[757] Increased growth hormone may be one normal physiological mechanism that accelerates muscle growth after exercise due to its anabolic action. Thus, the results of Chaikelis, which showed an increase in muscle strength after glycine,[749] may have been due to increased levels of growth hormone affecting a whole-body resistance training program, a situation not examined in the other reported studies on glycine and physical performance.[745,750-753]

In addition, glycine feeding with concurrent arginine feeding has been shown to significantly increase the rate of creatine synthesis.[536] This rate of synthesis would have resulted in a small body creatine pool increase, approximately 1 g/d. Whether this increase in creatine would improve physical performance is unknown.

No observable toxicity or ill effects have been noted after acute or chronic ingestion of large p.o. doses of glycine. Glycine is relatively inexpensive, readily available, and not unpalatable, having a sweet taste. Acute ingestion of large p.o. doses of glycine appears to stimulate release of growth hormone and increase creatine synthesis rates. Both of these attributes are desirable for persons undergoing progressive weight training. Aside from the suggestive report of Chaikelis,[749] no studies on effects of glycine on this type of training regime have been reported. Since growth hormone is also released after anaerobic or intermittent exercise,[758-765] glycine may possibly mimic or enhance this effect, leading to increased muscle mass formation over nonsupplemented controls when sufficient time is allowed. This hypothesis awaits testing. Glycine does not appear beneficial for endurance exercise, but studies measuring R, VO_2max, and other physiological parameters have not been performed.

No guidelines at this time are available for glycine supplementation as an ergogenic aid, although rather large doses (> 6 g/d) may be associated with physiological changes related to exercise enhancement.

VII. LYSINE

A doctoral thesis in 1960 reported on the physical performance test scores of sub-par college men after supplementation with lysine (790 mg) and a multiple vitamin.[766] Improvements were noted in both placebo and supplemented groups, but no differences between groups were seen. Oral administration of 1200 mg of L-lysine did not affect serum growth hormone levels in normal young males.[695]

VIII. ORNITHINE

A. SOMATOTROPIN RELEASE

Ornithine is similar to arginine and lysine in structure and function, with the exception that ornithine is not incorporated into proteins. Like arginine, ornithine infusion can release growth hormone in humans.[682,767,768] Doses are similar to arginine and well tolerated, with 12 g/m^2 producing fivefold increases in serum growth hormone in 45 min. However, clinical observations did not find increases in serum growth hormone 2 or 4 h after p.o. doses of 10 g of ornithine to normal subjects, although serum ornithine levels increased sevenfold.[769] It appears that testing of growth hormone levels at earlier times when a peak would be expected was not performed. Furthermore, after ornithine infusion, the peak of growth hormone returned to normal levels in 90 min.

Bucci et al. administered three different oral doses of ornithine·HCl on successive weekends to 12 bodybuilders after an overnight fast.[770] Doses were 40, 100, and 170 mg/kg of L-ornithine·HCl. Measurements of serum somatotropin levels at 0, 45, and 90 min after ornithine dosing found that 25% of subjects responded with a large increase in serum somatotropin at the two lower doses, and 50% of subjects responded at the highest dose, a significant difference. Serum ornithine levels increased in a dose-dependent manner up to four times initial levels,[770,771] suggesting that ornithine was the stimulus for somatotropin release. However, the highest ornithine dose was associated with osmotic diarrhea, making practical use of oral ornithine·HCl supplements for somatotropin release difficult. The three females responded at each dose, and were tested in pre-luteal phases of the menstrual cycle. Also, females did not exhibit osmotic diarrhea at high ornithine doses. These results suggest that oral ornithine should be studied in more detail in female strength athletes. The effect of oral ornithine on serum insulin levels was also studied.[772,773] No changes in serum insulin levels were seen, suggesting that oral ornithine is ineffective at stimulating insulin release.

B. OTHER PROPERTIES

Like arginine, ornithine is an amino acid involved in the urea cycle. In animal studies, ornithine (alone or in combination with other amino acids, especially aspartic acid) has been shown to reduce ammonia toxicity or blood levels in experimental situations.[705,715,716] The dipeptide, ornithine-aspartate, was shown to significantly reduce blood ammonia levels induced by exercise (swimming) in rats.[717] GPT enzyme and ATP levels were normalized by the dipeptide treatment. Administration of 6.4 g of p.o. ornithine to humans led to decreased blood urea levels, suggesting increased flux of the urea cycle.[774] Thus, ornithine may have practical ability to reduce exercise-induced ammonia levels and possibly delay fatigue.

Ornithine may offer ergogenic properties to athletes by yet another mechanism — polyamine synthesis.[773] Ornithine is the precursor for polyamine production, an important regulator of cell growth.[775,776] Addition of ornithine to human and rat liver cell cultures stimulated increased synthesis of albumin, an event mediated by polyamine synthesis.[777] Levels of serum ornithine found after oral supplementation[770,771,774,778] greatly exceeded culture concentrations found to stimulate albumin synthesis *in vitro*.

The study mentioned previously in the section on human studies with arginine employed a 1:1 mixture of arginine and ornithine (1 g each/d).[713] This study offers further evidence that oral ornithine supplements may possess ergogenic benefits for weightlifters.

Thus, oral ornithine supplementation has been demonstrated to affect physiological parameters that are of interest to athletes, especially weightlifters and bodybuilders. Whether a practical benefit from ornithine supplementation can be sustained in athletes remains to be determined.

Guidelines for use of ornithine are similar to arginine, and both amino acids can be regarded as interchangeable. However, at this time, guidelines on ornithine use are speculative only, and would amount to 2 to 20 g/d to possibly affect physiological parameters related to exercise performance in weightlifters.

IX. ORNITHINE-α-KETOGLUTARATE (OKG)

Ornithine-α-ketoglutarate (OKG) consists of two ornithine molecules bound to one α-ketoglutarate molecule, and has been in clinical use in Europe for a number of years.[779] For burns, trauma, sepsis, postsurgical repair, malnutrition, liver disease, renal disease, immunosuppression, and wound healing, at oral doses of 10 to 20 g/d, OKG has proven beneficial.[779,780] OKG appears to be a metabolic stimulus by a variety of mechanisms. Improvements in insulin and somatotropin secretion, increased protein synthesis, decreased protein catabolism, glutamine synthesis, polyamine synthesis, hydroxyproline synthesis (collagen), arginine and ketoacid effects have all been improved after OKG supplementation.[779,780] A potent action in protein metabolism has been observed, which may have application to strength athletes (weightlifters and bodybuilders), as well as to athletes wanting to recover from injuries as quickly as possible with the least loss of muscle mass. Use of OKG on athletes awaits further testing before any conclusions can be made about ergogenic effects for OKG. Safety and tolerability are well-documented.

X. TRYPTOPHAN

Oral administration of 5 g or more of tryptophan raised serum levels of growth hormone significantly in a majority of subjects.[781–785] However, side effects included drowsiness and mellow feelings,[781–785] quite in accord with the known properties of oral tryptophan.[786,787] Studies of athletes and growth hormone response to tryptophan have not been performed. It appears that tryptophan would not be a satisfactory candidate for stimulation of growth hormone release for several reasons. First, the number of responders is less than 100%, averaging 60%. Second, peak levels of growth hormone reached

10 to 15 ng/ml, which is much less than other forms of stimulation. Third, drowsiness may be detrimental to an athlete's performance. Fourth, tryptophan products sold to athletes contain only 250 or 500 mg per tablet or capsule, necessitating that they digest a large number of tablets per dose. Also, other amino acids are included in some products which would inhibit brain uptake and effect of tryptophan. Finally, tryptophan loading inhibits gluconeogenesis and urea metabolism.[788] Both processes are important for athletic performance.

Effects of acute doses of oral L-tryptophan (1200 mg in 24 h before testing) or a placebo on treadmill performance and nociception were reported in a randomized, double-blind, crossover study.[789] Total exercise time and total work load performed were greatly increased (49%) after tryptophan administration, and ratings of perceived exertion were lowered. Results suggest that oral tryptophan administration may have affected endogenous endorphin/enkephalin levels to provide an increased pain tolerance, allowing for greater work performance.

However, events in 1989 have made purified tryptophan unavailable for public consumption. Outbreaks of Eosinophilia-Myalgia Syndrome (EMS) were traced to a contaminated batch of L-tryptophan from one Japanese manufacturer, used for dietary supplements, infant formulas, and intravenous infusions.[790–793] Over 15,000 cases of EMS have been reported, with 27 associated deaths. One or more tryptophan dimers (formed from tryptophan and acetaldehyde) were accidentally produced by a modified production method, and these dimers have been implicated as the cause of EMS outbreaks.[792,793] The Food and Drug Administration recalled and banned sales of tryptophan in supplement form in 1989, and recalled infant formulas and intravenous solutions in 1990.[792] At this time, since tryptophan is an indispensable amino acid, purified tryptophan can be used to fortify protein products, but pure tryptophan cannot be sold. There is some evidence that very large doses of tryptophan may have the potential to form toxic dimers from physiological exposure to aldehydes, which would argue against taking large doses of tryptophan for long time periods.[793] Thus, use of tryptophan by athletes in doses necessary for the effects observed in the studies cited above is not possible at this time.

XI. SUMMARY OF AMINO ACID ERGOGENIC PROPERTIES

Only a few of the known amino acids have been tested to modulate responses of interest for exercise (see Table 1). Almost no data on normal, exercising humans are available; thus, no conclusions about effects of individual amino acids on physical performance, with the exception of glycine, can be made. Further testing using adequate doses and times of administration to athletes may confirm or deny the benefits seen for some clinical conditions by administration of arginine, aspartate, glutamate, glycine, ornithine, OKG, and BCAA. Potential uses for other singular amino acids may also be discovered.

TABLE 1

Ergogenic Effects in Humans after Oral Dosing with Single Amino Acids

Amino acid	Daily dose		Findings related to exercise	Ref.
Arginine	5 g, 250 mg/kg	↑	somatotropin release upon stimulus	692, 693
	4 g	↑	creatine stores	536
Arginine pyroglutamate/ Lysine	1.2 g each	↑	serum somatotropin	695
Arginine/Ornithine	1 g each	↑	body fat & weight loss during weightlifting program	713
Aspartate Salts	7–10 g	↑	time to exhaustion, untrained subjects	476–478, 480
Glycine	6.8–30 g	↑	serum somatotropin	754, 756
	6 g	↑	muscular strength	749
Ornithine	170 mg/kg	↑	serum somatotropin (diarrhea side effects)	770
Ornithine α-Ketoglutarate	10–20 g	↑	serum somatotropin & insulin protein synthesis, anabolism	779, 780
Tryptophan	≥ 5 g	↑	serum somatotropin	781–785
	1.2 g	↑	work load & exercise time	789

Chapter 7

SPECIFIC COMBINATIONS OF NUTRIENTS

I. MIXTURES OF MICRONUTRIENTS

An almost limitless number of possible combinations of ergogenic aids is imaginable. Many combinations have been or are currently being marketed. Obviously, the ability to design or market combinations is far easier than to test them rigorously. Thus, reports in peer-reviewed literature concerning ergogenic effects of combinations are few.

A combination of citrated caffeine (300 mg), sodium citrate (1000 mg), sodium phosphate (500 mg), dextrose (370 mg), ascorbic acid (75 mg), and thiamine (5 mg) was administered daily for 10 d in a double-blind study by Arterbury in 1971, as cited by Williams.[794] Strength, endurance, and recovery were not affected by the supplement, as was determined by tests on a cable tensiometer and arm ergometer.

A combination of high dose B vitamins, vitamin C, free-form amino acids, arginine, ornithine, γ-oryzanol, octacosanol, chlorophyll, coenzyme Q_{10}, and glandular tablets was given daily to 13 male college athletes for 8 weeks.[795] Compared to 20 controls, supplemented subjects consistently lost body fat (−3.4%) and increased muscle girth measurements. A placebo effect could not be ruled out since the study was not blind.

A supplement containing B vitamins, vitamin A, vitamin C, calcium, magnesium, potassium, phosphate, amino acids, nucleic acids, and rutin was given for 20 d to 7 males.[796] A submaximal step test was used to measure performance, and a reduction of heart rate during exercise from 134 to 111 bpm was found. However, since supplements were given after a control period, a training effect cannot be ruled out, leaving the results equivocal.[796]

A multivitamin mixture containing vitamins A, C, D, B_1, B_2, B_6, B_{12}, niacinamide, pantothenate, and folate was administered to college males for 11 weeks.[766] No differences in test scores of physical performance were found between a placebo group and the supplemented group.

Twenty well-trained, male runners were administered either a placebo or a commercial multivitamin/multimineral supplement for 4 weeks.[797] No effects on VO_2max, muscle glycogen depletion, serum FFA levels, serum glucose levels, or serum lactate levels during or after 50 min treadmill runs (65 to 70% of VO_2max) were seen. Levels of B vitamins ranged from 15 to 21 mg, while other vitamins and trace minerals were near or below USRDA values. Compared to studies in Table 2 of Chapter 3, these doses of B vitamins appear to be insufficient to elicit ergogenic effects in normal individuals.

Likewise, another long-term, double-blind, crossover, placebo-controlled study with 30 male runners found no influences on measurements of exercise performance from "...a comprehensive multivitamin and mineral supplement. ..."[798] However, the composition of the mixture was not stated; therefore, no comparisons to Table 2 (Chapter 3) or other studies can be made.

Yet another placebo-controlled study measured performances in maximal cycle ergometry speed, vertical jump, and 10-yd sprint times after physical education students and football players were given an unspecified dose of an unnamed, but popular, multiple vitamin/mineral product, as cited by Williams.[199] Contents of the product were not disclosed. Again, no comparisons to other studies or Table 2 (Chapter 3) can be made.

The ergogenic effects of Enerzyme® products Race Caps and Enduro Caps, dietary supplements providing vitamin E succinate, inosine, coenzyme Q_{10}, magnesium glycerol phosphate, and cytochrome c, in doses between 10 to 100 mg each, were studied in 22 collegiate swimmers and 8 cross-country runners for 6 weeks with a double-blind study design.[799] Performance times for a 1000 yd swim or progressive treadmill test to VO_2max were not significantly different between supplemented and control groups. Comparison to other studies would also predict the lack of ergogenic effect for doses given in this study, even if only vitamin E was considered.

Ergogenic effects of a vitamin/electrolyte/carbohydrate drink were studied in 12 males by measurements during a submaximal cycle ergometer test.[800] The drink was composed of 10 to 25 mg each of vitamins B_1, B_2, B_3, B_5, and B_6; 500 mg vitamin C; 50 mg vitamin E; 250 mg calcium; 170 mg magnesium; 100 mg potassium; 1.08 g of phosphorus (as phosphate), and 3.8 g of complex carbohydrates. A dose of 1.2 l was split in four equal doses and given before and during 120 min of exercise. Work efficiency improved, and heart rate decreased, compared to a control period of water intake. Unfortunately, conclusions are suspect since no statistical analysis was reported.[199]

The availability of specific nutrient combinations has grown to the point where over a hundred brands have between one and several dozen products marketed specifically for exercise and sports applications. Product sophistication continues to outpace any possibility of definitive testing, much less of preliminary studies. The demand for new products is fueled by the willingness of the public to try products that are usually untested and based on hypothetical mechanisms. Certainly, a placebo response is gained with indiscriminate use of various nutritional supplement products, and this response alone may well be sufficient to encourage continued usage and improvements in exercise performance. Whether commercially available products have effects beyond placebo responses is still largely untested.

II. SPECIFIC MACRONUTRIENT MANIPULATION

Another category of combinations of nutritional ergogenic aids is dietary manipulation of macronutrient compositions to accentuate certain hormone levels, which, in turn, will affect exercise metabolism. An example is the BIOSYN system developed by Barry Sears, Ph.D.[171] A comprehensive and simple diet program incorporating everyday foods is based on the relationship between insulin and glucagon, levels of which can be influenced by food intake. Recent research shows that extended, high insulin output from constant, high-carbohydrate diets (such as those recommended for glycogen supercompensation) depresses fatty acid output,[801] inhibits somatotropin release,[802] and promotes storage of excess calories as fat. Glucagon is a mobilization hormone that produces glucose from glycogen and fatty acids from stored body fat.[803] Exercise inhibits insulin secretion[804] and stimulates glucagon secretion.[805,806] Thus, a balance between insulin and glucagon that safely favors release of body fat stores while maintaining lean muscle mass has important ergogenic effects while consuming fewer total calories than other diets. The key to balancing insulin and glucagon release is to consume *at each feeding* a protein to carbohydrate ratio of 0.6 to 0.7 (grams or calories). Thus, a typical dietary analysis would reveal a diet consisting of 30% protein, 40% carbohydrates, and 30% fat. Total calories are adjusted to prevent hunger or weight gain. This dietary plan has been used with success by various sports associations, including the NFLPA.

Chapter 8

DIETARY SUBSTANCES NOT REQUIRED IN HUMAN METABOLISM

I. ALCOHOL (ETHANOL)

This section will only briefly review effects of alcohol on performance, since alcohol (ethanol) is legally a drug and may cause disqualification in certain athletic competitions. Ethanol is a normal bodily and dietary component and thus cannot be ignored.

According to several excellent reviews, the predominant effects of ethanol are psychological.[807] Small amounts of ethanol can reduce tension and insecurity, leading to increased self-confidence and thus improved performance in some individuals.[807] Both stimulant and tranquilizing effects may be advantageous to certain individuals. Larger doses of alcohol (0.040 to 0.075% blood levels) are definitely a detriment to motor performance, judgment, information processing, reaction time, hand-eye coordination, accuracy, balance, steadiness, and complex coordination skills.[807] Blood alcohol levels of 0.10% or greater are considered in legal terms as intoxication. Thus, overwhelming evidence conclusively demonstrates that ethanol intoxication adversely affects physical performance.

Ethanol has been shown to have no effect or a slightly adverse effect on tests of muscular strength.[807] Likewise, ethanol has not affected VO2max, heart rate, stroke volume, blood pressure, or peak lactate levels.[807] Ethanol doses offer increased risks of hypothermia in cold temperatures and dehydration.[807]

In general, no harm or detriment to performance has been shown after moderate ethanol consumption (one drink per day).[807] One drink is defined as 12 oz of beer, 4 oz (one glass) of wine, or 1 oz of 100% proof hard liquor. Excessive consumption will lead to decreases in performance and health.

II. CAFFEINE

A. INTRODUCTION

Caffeine has been used since the Stone Age as a stimulant.[807] Major dietary sources are coffee, tea, chocolate, colas, and several herbs which constitute important dietary items for most cultures.[807-809] Theophylline and theobromine are other methylxanthines found in significant amounts in teas and chocolates.[807-811] Caffeine is also present in many nonprescription medications.[808,809] Daily intake of caffeine from dietary sources can range from 0 to over 1 g/d.[808-810] Widespread availability, low cost, and social acceptance have allowed caffeine to be well studied. Caffeine has been shown to stimulate neurons, the central nervous system, cardiac muscles, diuresis, epinephrine release and actions, lipolysis of adipose tissue increasing serum FFA levels,

83

relaxation of smooth muscle, and gastric acid secretion.[807,809] Several of these effects have been postulated to improve physical performance.

B. HUMAN STUDIES

Use of caffeine to enhance human performance has been examined since 1893.[811] Unfortunately, most studies prior to 1960 are difficult to analyze owing to low subject numbers, uncontrolled designs, inaccurate or imprecise performance measurements, or lack of metabolic substrate measurements.[807,810,811] Research during the 1960s found that caffeine had no effect on treadmill run times to exhaustion[812,813] or on isometric strength.[814] More recent research has produced studies that have revealed further the effects of caffeine on physical performance. Table 1 summarizes the results of 15 studies on the effects of caffeine on metabolism and performance during exercise.[93,815-829] All studies cited used either a single-blind (6/15) or double-blind (9/15) design. Doses of caffeine were comparable for all studies, corresponding to an average of two to three cups of coffee (200 to 300 mg).

Caffeine was administered 60 min before exercise in all but one study, compatible with the known absorption and clearance of caffeine.[830] Except for one study on cross-country ski races, all studies employed either cycle ergometry (10/15) or treadmill running (4/15). Length of exercise times of greater than 30 min were associated with significant changes in performance or metabolic measurements in caffeine-treated groups (8/10), while short-term maximal exercise was not (0/3).

The issue of tolerance to caffeine was not addressed in 12/15 studies, although most studies required subjects to abstain from caffeine for 8 to 48 h. Habitual caffeine users develop a tolerance to its effects.[831-834] Caffeine withdrawal necessitates a 3 to 4 d washout period.[829,831-834] Fisher et al. studied untrained women habituated to caffeine before and after a 4-d withdrawal period.[829] Significant changes in metabolism and performance after caffeine administration were seen only after the withdrawal period, indicating caffeine tolerance decreases the effect of supplemental caffeine on exercise. Toner et al. studied eight subjects and found that the only two subjects who did not show an increase in VO$_2$max were the only two subjects who consumed caffeine (100 mg/d).[822] Furthermore, the lack of effect found for caffeine on maximal muscular performance of 14 female college students may have been due to a slight tolerance as discussed by Perkins and Williams.[815] Thus, the lack of caffeine intake history or consideration may account for some of the variability between studies listed in Table 1. The caffeine intake history of subjects in future studies should be recorded, since even habituation to 100 mg/d (equivalent to two soft drinks or one cup of coffee) may obscure results, and caffeine-containing products are commonly consumed.

C. FACTORS AFFECTING CAFFEINE RESEARCH

Three studies examined various doses of caffeine, and none found a dose response.[815,823,824] The effect of training was compared in two

TABLE 1
Summary of Experimental Variables and Results from 15 Studies on Effects of Caffeine on Exercise Performance Metabolism

Subject no./ gender	Avg. age (yr)	Training status	Caffeine status	Caffeine dose	Exp. design	Type of exercise	Performance changes	Metabolic changes	Ref.
14/female	22	Un-trained	Possibly tolerant	0,4,7,10 mg/kg	Double-blind	Cycle ergometer (maximal)	Time to exhaustion, NS	HR, RPE, NS	815
7/male 2/female	22	Competitive cyclists	NR	330 mg	Blind	Cycle ergometer (maximal)	Time to exhaustion, increased (90 vs. 76 min)	FFA, glycerol, fat oxidation increased; R decreased; HR, VO₂, RPE, lactate, glucose, triglycerides, carbohydrate oxidation NS	816
7/male 2/female	23	Competitive cyclists	NR	250 mg	Blind	Cycle ergometer (submaximal)	Total work increased (117,016 vs. 108,984 kph)	VO₂, FFA, O₂ pulse, fat oxidation increased; HR, R, RPE, glycerol, glucose, insulin, carbohydrate oxidation NS	817
7/male	26	Competitive cyclists	NR	5 mg/kg	Blind	Cycle ergometer (submaximal)	Total work, NS	R, carbohydrate oxidation, muscle glycogen, utilization decreased; FFA, muscle triglyceride utilization, fat oxidation increased; VO₂, lactate, glycerol, glucose NS	818
7/NR	NR	Competitive cyclists	NR	5 mg/kg	Double-blind	Cycle ergometer (maximal)	Time to exhaustion, NS	Anerobic threshold, VO₂max NS	819
5/female 8/male	20–30	Competitive cross-country skiers	NR	6 mg/kg	Double-blind	High-altitude (2900 m) cross-country ski races	Race times decreased (99 vs. 102 min)	RPE NS	820

TABLE 1 (continued)
Summary of Experimental Variables and Results from 15 Studies on Effects of Caffeine on Exercise Performance Metabolism

Subject no./ gender	Avg. age (yr)	Training status	Caffeine status	Caffeine dose	Exp. design	Type of exercise	Performance changes	Metabolic changes	Ref.
4/female 10/male	20–30	Competitive cross-country skiers	NR	6 mg/kg	Double-blind	Low-altitude (300 m) cross-country ski races	Race times decreased (99 vs. 101 min)	RPE NS	820
5/male	26–30	NR	NR	4 mg/kg	Blind	Cycle ergometer (submaximal) in cold (5°C)	NR	VO_2, VE increased; R, rectal temperature decreased; HR, FFA, NS	821
5/male	26–30	NR	NR	4 mg/kg	Blind	Cycle ergometer (submaximal)	NR	VO_2, VE increased; R decreased; HR, FFA, rectal temperature NS	821
8/male	28	4 trained 4 untrained	Naive (<100 mg/dl)	350 mg	Double-blind	Cycle ergometer (maximal)	Time to exhaustion	HR, VO_2 increased; VE, R, cardiac output, arteriovenous O_2 difference, systole volume NS	822
4/female 4/male	NR	NR	None in 48 h	0,2,2, 4,4,8.8 mg/kg	Double-blind	Treadmill run (maximal)	Time to exhaustion, increased (4.4 mg/kg)	Lactate, glycerol increased; HR, R, RPE, FFA NS	823
5/male	NR	Trained (32 mi/w)	NR	0,5,9 mg/kg	Double-blind	Treadmill run (submaximal)	NR	Glucose, FFA increased; R, lactate, glycerol NS	824

Subjects	Training status	Age	Dose		Design	Exercise	Performance	Results	Ref.
5/male	Un-trained	NR	NR		Double-blind	Treadmill run (submaximal)		Lactate, FFA, glycerol, glucose increased; R NS	824
10/male	5 trained, 5 un-trained	NR	0,5,9 mg/kg		Double-blind	Treadmill run (submaximal)		Trained vs. untrained: R, FFA, lactate, glycerol, glucose significantly different	824
7/male	Trained	NR	5 mg/kg		Blind	Cycle ergometer (maximal)	Time to exhaustion, NS	FFA, glycerol increased; lactate NS	825
15/female 13/male	Active college students	23	300 mg		Double-blind	Cycle ergometer (maximal)	Time to exhaustion, NS	HR, VO_2, VE, R, RPE, NS	826
9/male	Mara-thoners	30	400 mg		Double-blind	Treadmill run (submaximal)		VE, lactate increased; HR, VO_2, R, RPE, FFA, glucose, triglycerides NS	827
8/male	Un-trained	28	5 mg/kg		Blind	Cycle ergometer (maximal)	Maximal work rate, NS	Lactate, O_2 pulse increased; HR decreased; VO_2, VE, R, NS	828
6/female	Un-trained	21–34	788 mg/d tolerant	None in 8 h	Double-blind	Treadmill run (submaximal)		HR, VO_2, R, RPE, FFA, lactate, dopamine, norepinephrine, NS	
6/female	Un-trained	21–34	5 mg/kg (Withdrawn)	None in 4 d	Double-blind	Treadmill run (submaximal)		VO_2, FFA, dopamine, norepinephrine increased; HR, R decreased; RPE, lactate NS	830

Note: NS, Not significant; NR, not reported; HR, heart rate; RPE, rating of perceived exertion; R, respiratory quotient; FFA, serum free fatty acids; VO_2, oxygen uptake; VO_2max, maximal oxygen capacity; VE, lung ventilation.

studies.[822,824] Toner et al. found no differences in responses between four competitive cyclists and four untrained men,[822] while Knapik et al. found significant effects from caffeine in untrained but not trained subjects.[824] Thus, training status was not correlated with responses to caffeine. Six studies utilized trained athletes, five utilized untrained subjects, and four did not report on the training status of subjects. Five of eight studies with trained athletes showed changes after caffeine supplementation, while four of seven studies with untrained athletes showed change.

Another experimental variable on the metabolic effects of caffeine is the state of body carbohydrate stores and ingestion. Weir and co-workers recently discovered that a high carbohydrate diet for 3 d (analogous to glycogen supercompensation) and a high carbohydrate prevent meal prevented the expected rise in serum FFA levels during exercise.[835] Thus, nutritional status of subjects may affect results of previous studies.

D. PHYSIOLOGICAL EFFECTS OF CAFFEINE

Caffeine ingestion increased plasma FFA concentration significantly when compared to control, exercised groups in six of nine studies. Only one study using trained marathon runners and two studies that did not report the training status of subjects did not show increases. Tolerance to caffeine did not result in a significant increase of FFA levels by caffeine.[829] Plasma glycerol levels were significantly increased in four of seven studies, with all three studies using untrained subjects reporting increases. Plasma glucose values were elevated in one of five studies. Lactate levels increased in four of nine studies, with three of five studies using untrained subjects responding. Glucose and FFA values were both increased simultaneously in only one of five studies. Lactate and FFA levels were both increased in two studies (untrained subjects), while four studies showed increases in FFA but not lactate (three with trained subjects), and two studies showed increased lactate but not FFA. Thus, a consensus of research shows that caffeine usually causes an increase in lipolytic products (FFA and glycerol) over the effect of exercise alone, but glycogenolytic products, glucose and lactate, may be elevated independently of lipolytic status. Caffeine induced sparing of muscle glycogen (42%) while decreasing muscle triglyceride by 105% greater than controls in trained subjects undergoing submaximal exercise in one report.[818] Although carbohydrate utilization was depressed in the caffeine group (52 g compared to 79 g), fat oxidation was increased (21 g compared to 14 g), and total work output was similar for both groups. Two other reports using the same subjects reported no differences in carbohydrate utilization, but large increases in fat oxidation (31 and 107% above control values) and in total work output.[816,817]

Heart rate (HR) was increased in one study, decreased in two, and did not change in seven reports when compared to placebo group. Oxygen uptake (VO_2) was improved in four of the studies, while the respiratory exchange ratio (R) showed a decrease in four of eleven reports. Ratings of perceived exertion (RPE) did not change in eight studies measuring RPE. Thus, beneficial effects of caffeine on physiological parameters relevant to endurance were not found in a majority of studies. Correlation of increases in physiologic parameters with metabolic changes were seen in six of ten studies.

E. PERFORMANCE EFFECTS OF CAFFEINE

Time to exhaustion or work output was improved in caffeine-treated groups in four of ten studies. All four positive studies also showed improvements in metabolic or physiologic measurements. Three of six studies reporting no significant difference in performance did show significant changes in metabolic or physiologic measurements. Large variability in performance among subjects was noted in the studies showing improvement. Essig et al. reported a range of increases in cycle ergometer times to exhaustion of 0 to 80%,[818] while Butts and Crowell noted one subject improved her cycling time by 49%, rendering significance to the group cycling time average.[826] Perhaps ratios of fast and slow twitch fibers also affect results, a variable not addressed in any caffeine study. Responses of mouse soleus (slow) and gastrocnemius (fast) muscles showed large differences when exposed to caffeine *in vitro*.[836] Thus, muscle fiber composition differences could add to the variability seen among studies in responses to caffeine.

Nine recent studies found significant increases in performance and/or significant changes in metabolic parameters,[837-845] while one study was equivocal,[846] and one study found no effects on performance.[847] Metabolites of caffeine (paraxanthine) may account for caffeine effects.[812,845] Finally, reaction times and movement times after moderate (300 mg) but not high (600 mg) doses of caffeine were found to be improved.[841]

One interesting notion that has not been fully tested in humans yet is the use of caffeine with aerobic exercise to reduce body fat quicker than exercise alone. In one study, male rats subjected to exercise and caffeine did not show a difference in total carcass body fat over exercised rats (5.4 compared to 6.7%).[848] Epididymal fat pads weighed less from the caffeine group, but the difference was not significant. The same author had earlier shown significant decreases in epididymal fat pad weight, retroperitoneal fat pad weight, and epididymal fat cell size in rats exercised with caffeine compared to exercise only.[849] With aerobic fitness programs in order to lose weight (body fat) maintaining popularity, especially among females, studies concerning the effects of caffeine on body fat loss would be helpful.

Also, excessive amounts of caffeine (over five cups of coffee before a competition) may produce a urinary level sufficient for disqualification in events that test for doping.[850] Serum levels of caffeine above 5 mcg/ml are associated with respiratory stimulation.[850] These levels are easily achieved with ingestion of 200 to 300 mg of caffeine.[823] With unacceptable urine levels of caffeine set at 15 mcg/ml,[850] great caution is required for athletes undergoing doping analysis and using caffeine.

Another potential drawback of caffeine is toxicity. Caffeine has known diuretic abilities,[807-811] a condition which may be deleterious if exercise is conducted in hot, humid weather. Caffeine in large doses can also produce delirium, hallucinations, anxiety, and memory impairment during conditions of prolonged competitive stress.[851] Insomnia, heart arrhythmias, and gastric upset have been reported at doses of 200 to 500 mg in some individuals.[807]

F. SUMMARY AND GUIDELINES

In summary, caffeine can spare muscle glycogen and increase oxidation of intramuscular fat in some caffeine-naive, trained individuals, leading to improvement in performance or work output during long-term endurance running or cycling. Untrained individuals usually show increased hydrolysis and utilization of glycogen with caffeine or exercise rather than a sparing effect, regardless of lipolytic status. Caffeine does not appear to benefit short-term, maximal exercise, although recent studies using weightlifters have not been reported. Thus, caffeine appears to enhance performance over a placebo effect in some persons, but in less than a majority. Since caffeine is inexpensive and easy to procure, persons may determine for themselves whether caffeine would be useful, although placebo effects must be accounted for.

Guidelines for caffeine ingestion to enhance endurance performance in trained, non-coffee-drinking individuals are 200 to 300 mg, equivalent to two to three cups of coffee (fresh-brewed) 1 h before an event. Proper hydration is important to prevent possible diuretic effects of caffeine. The suggested doses are below those levels of caffeine that are unacceptable to drug testing authorities in sports competitions.

III. FERULATES

Ferulic acid is a common phenolic acid found in almost every plant.[852] Gamma oryzanol, a ferulate ester of sterols found in rice bran, has also been the subject of studies. Gamma oryzanol is mostly converted to ferulic acid during digestion.[852] Ferulic acid closely mimics the structure of normetanephrine, the primary metabolite of norepinephrine.[852] Animal studies have found that ferulate administration can mimic effects of increased hypothalamic norepinephrine,[852] such as stimulation of somatotropin synthesis by the pituitary.[853–855] Infusion of 100 or 500 mg of ferulic acid (0.3 mg/kg) into heifers elevated serum somatotropin levels significantly.[856] Other pituitary hormones were generally not affected.[852–856]

In addition, ferulic acid is a potent antioxidant, with activity similar to vitamin E both *in vitro*[857–859] and *in vivo*.[860,861] Oral supplementation of 40 women with elevated serum lipid peroxide levels with 300 mg of gamma oryzanol for 4 to 8 weeks led to significant decreases to normal levels.[862] Thus, ferulates measurable antioxidant activity after oral supplementation in humans.

Because of potential effects on somatotropin and antioxidant effects, first gamma oryzanol and then ferulic acid were studied in weightlifters for possible ergogenic effects. A series of small, poorly controlled studies found significant increases in lean body mass, significant decreases in body fat, significant increases in strength, improved recovery from workouts, and less post-exercise muscle soreness in supplemented subjects, compared to control subjects.[852]

A double-blind, multi-center study administered a placebo (n=4) or 30 mg of trans-ferulic acid (n=6) daily for 8 weeks to trained weightlifters. [863,864] Body weight increased significantly for supplemented subjects (+1.9 kg), but not for placebo subjects (–0.6 kg). Strength as measured by one-repetition maximum lift for the shoulder press was significantly increased in the supplemented group compared to the control group (+5.3 vs. –0.3 kg). Strength changes for leg press and chest press one-repetition maxima showed trends towards increases in the supplemented group. Dietary intakes were not different between the two groups. Thus, supplemental ferulate appeared to augment some aspects of resistance training.

Another double-blind, randomized crossover study measured stress hormone levels in serum before and after strenuous exercise in six well-trained male endurance runners, with ferulate intake (50 mg/d for 3 weeks) the major variable.[865] Resting hormone levels were not influenced by ferulate supplementation. After exercise, significant increases from resting levels for cortisol, testosterone, and beta endorphin were seen during both placebo and supplemented periods. However, beta endorphin levels during the supplemented period were significantly greater than the placebo period. These results support a hypothalamic effect on catecholamine neurotransmitters suggested by animal research.

Thus, two recent double-blind studies have found ergogenic abilities for ferulic acid, a common plant compound. Ferulates are the only nutritional compound to date that have shown effects on endorphins in athletes. It is conceivable that higher levels of endorphins released during exercise may lead to reduced perception of fatigue, allowing exercise to be continued slightly longer than it otherwise would have. If this effect were maintained for an extended training period, nonspecific enhancement of training effects might result that would hasten improvements in exercise performance. Safety and commercial availability argue for further testing of ferulates as ergogenic aids.

Although studies suggest that ferulate supplementation appears promising as a possible nutritional alternative to anabolic steroid use for weightlifters, further research is necessary to define potential dose-response effects. Thus, guidelines for ferulate or gamma oryzanol supplementation would be premature. At this time, doses of 50 to 300 mg/d appear safe.

IV. GELATIN

When glycine was found to be a precursor for creatine, as well as being of potential benefit for relief of muscular fatigue,[737,748] administration of gelatin was postulated as a potential ergogenic aid. Gelatin is protein derived from animal collagen containing 25% glycine.[752] Gelatin is an incomplete protein, meaning it lacks sufficient essential amino acid content to become the sole source of nitrogen intake for humans.

Three initial studies around 1940 found enormous increases in work capacity of men (but not of women) on cycle ergometers,[866] and in work capacity of men and women (trained and untrained).[867,868] However, due to inadequacies in experimental design, these studies actually measured training effects. Thus, they cannot be regarded as conclusive.

Meanwhile, nine separate studies found no benefit from gelatin administration.[750,751,869-875] Most of these studies employed an experimental design that was not biased by training or psychological effects. Subjects included male and female athletes that ran, cycled, swam, or lifted weights. Measurements of delayed muscle soreness, race times from 0.5 to 1.5 m, efficiency of grade walking, cycle ergometry, swim times for 60 to 100-yd races, number of wall weight pulls, attempts to break previous personal records for weightlifting, and arm ergograph work were analyzed. Doses of gelatin ranged from 30 to 60 g daily for long periods of time (weeks and months). Thus, 7.5 to 14 g additional of glycine were added to each subject's daily diet. However, one factor not considered by these studies is the poor absorption of hydroxyproline-containing peptides (some with glycine) from normal digestion of gelatin.[876] In view of the lack of effect on the above-mentioned parameters, gelatin is not an ergogenic aid for exercise or sports.

V. GINSENG

A. INTRODUCTION

For centuries, the root of the plant *Panax ginseng* has been used as a prophylactic tonic to reduce fatigue in Oriental cultures. Currently 8.5×10^6 lb/yr of ginseng root, with a value of $1 billion, is marketed worldwide.[877] Active ingredients have been characterized as over 20 structurally similar steroid glycosides (saponins) named ginsenosides.[877] This mixture comprises 1 to 2% of *P. ginseng*, being variable from plant to plant and even more variable in commercial preparations, some containing no ginsenosides.[877] Thus, the form of ginseng used in studies on exercise performance is a major uncontrolled variable.

Various extracts of ginseng root containing ginsenosides have been shown to spare glycogen utilization and increase oxidation of fatty acids as shown by reduced lactate and pyruvate and increased glucose levels in exercised rats.[878-882] Increased endurance or reduction of fatigue in exercised animals has been seen following oral or injected administration of ginsenosides.[880,883-885] In addition, oral ginsenoside treatments have been shown to have anabolic actions in animals, as shown by increases in DNA, RNA, and protein synthesis.[880,886] Thus, a rationale for use to enhance endurance performance and promote recovery from exercise by administration of ginsenosides has been established in animal studies.

B. HUMAN STUDIES

Studies with human subjects have failed to find ergogenic effects of 200 or 2000 mg of ginseng root given daily for 4 to 9 weeks.[887-889] Lactate, glucose,

FFA, glycerol, insulin, growth hormone, VO_2max, heart rate, RPE, and run times showed no differences from control groups. However, compared to animal studies, very small doses of ginsenosides were used. Approximately 30 mg of ginsenosides (0.4 mg/kg) from 2000 mg ginseng root (1.5% ginsenosides)[889] per person per day were administered, whereas animal studies used up to 200 mg/kg of ginsenoside fractions.

One abstract reported improved VO_2max, improved speed of recovery (post-exercise heart rate), and improved reaction time after ginseng administration.[890] However, no doses were reported. A recent study compared placebo, Chinese ginseng (Panax species), and Russian ginseng *(Eleutherococcus senticosus)* supplementation in a randomized, double-blind study at intake levels of 1 g/d.[890] It was found that Chinese ginseng, but not Russian ginseng, was associated with a significantly increased VO_2max when compared to the placebo group. Both ginsengs were associated with increased pectoral and quadriceps strength when compared to placebos.

In a double-blind study, 50 healthy male sports teachers (21 to 47 years) were given a placebo or a supplement containing ginseng extract, dimethylaminoethanol bitartrate (DMAE), vitamins, minerals, and trace elements for 6 weeks.[891] Physical performance was assessed by progressively increasing workloads on a treadmill. Total work load and VO_2max were significantly greater for the supplemented group. For identical workloads, plasma lactate, ventilation, carbon dioxide production, and heart rate during exercise were significantly lower for supplemented subjects. Effects were most pronounced in subjects with VO_2max <60 ml/kg/min. The results indicate that work capacity was increased by improved muscular oxygenation. These reports offer the first evidence that ginseng may be an ergogenic aid for endurance athletes and strength athletes.

C. SUMMARY AND GUIDELINES

It is also known that American ginseng *(P. quinquefolium)* and red ginseng (steam-treated for preservation) are not comparable in ginsenoside activity to *P ginseng* ginsenosides.[892] In addition, thermolability of ginsenosides has been reported.[877] Thus, great caution must be used by both researchers and consumers when ginseng products are chosen for experimentation or use. A "standardized" ginseng extract with respect to ginsenoside content is currently being offered, but no human exercise studies using this product have been reported. Whether the effects seen in animal studies from large doses of ginsenosides are reproducible in humans is unknown. It is known that small amounts of some ginseng root preparations do not enhance aerobic performance, and one human study using large doses of Chinese ginseng found some ergogenic benefits.

Guidelines for use of ginseng as an ergogenic aid must consider the ginsenoside content in any ginseng preparation. Unless ginsenoside content is accurately known, guidelines would be subject to great error. It does appear that, for ginseng to have any promise as an ergogenic aid, doses of 1 g/d or more of a standardized, ginsenoside-rich extract are necessary.

VI. OCTACOSANOL AND WHEAT GERM OIL

A. INTRODUCTION

Effects of wheat germ oil (WGO) as prepared by Viobin Corporation have been studied for a number of years by Cureton. While the components of WGO used by Cureton were never completely characterized, linoleic acid (in triglyceride form), vitamin E, octacosanol, choline, and other vitamins and minerals are known to be present.[307] Other compounds found in grain germ oils such as sterols are probably present, and a known amount of ferulate (340 mg/100 g) is also present.[893]

B. HUMAN STUDIES

Cureton reported many ergogenic effects of WGO from results of 42 studies with 894 subjects compiled in a book in 1972.[307] Many experimental results appear only in this book. Placebo groups were utilized, incorporating isocaloric, devitaminized (or with vitamin E added) oils or lard. Cardiovascular performance, muscular endurance, and strength were measured. Improvements in endurance and reaction times were reported.[307,894,895] Cureton states that, at doses equivalent to 4 ml/d, 4 to 5 weeks are necessary before statistical significance is achieved.[307] Furthermore, the "active principle" of WGO was shown to be octacosanol, a long-chain waxy alcohol found in a concentration of 0.011% in WGO.[307] Although a physiological mechanism of action for octacosanol or WGO has not been found, Cureton attributed its effects to increased oxygen transport.

Other investigators have found WGO or octacosanol improved conditioned reflexes, but not oxygen transport or endurance.[896,897] Russian studies summarized by Brozek[896] even stated that Americans overemphasized oxygen transport compared to nervous reflexes for WGO. Octacosanol (1000 mcg/d for 8 weeks) was administered in double-blind fashion to 16 students.[897] Reaction time to visual stimuli and grip strength increased significantly as analyzed by ANOVA. Auditory reaction times improved, but did not reach statistical significance. Chest strength and cycle ergometer endurance were not affected by octacosanol.

Other reports did not find an effect of WGO on electrocardiographic T-wave amplitude, as cited by Williams.[794,898] T-wave amplitude is still not substantiated as a determinant of physical fitness. Unpublished theses by Coulson and Fulton, cited by Williams,[794] also did not find ergogenic benefits of WGO. Coulson found that 4 weeks of WGO administration did not augment the effects of training for 36 lacrosse team members as measured by exhaustive cycle ergometer trials. Fulton found that junior high school athletes given WGO for 12 weeks did not show improvements over placebo and control groups for arm strength, speed, endurance, and body weight changes.

Animal studies were equally ambiguous. Both increases in swim times[899] and no effects on swim times[900,901] have been reported for both WGO and octacosanol.

C. SUMMARY AND GUIDELINES

Thus, a consensus of results indicated that WGO and/or octacosanol probably do not improve endurance capacity reproducibly. Rather, octacosanol may improve neuro-muscular functions such as reaction time. These findings are compatible with clinical benefits found after octacosanol or WGO supplementation to patients with nervous disorders.[902-905] It appears that a possible mechanism of action for octacosanol could be stabilization of cell membranes, particularly nerve cell membranes, by virtue of its molecular size and shape.

Guidelines for octacosanol use need further refinement. However, a preliminary suggestion has been made that 1000 to 10,000 µg/d of octacosanol taken over a period greater than 6 weeks may be helpful for sports where reaction time is critical (baseball, football, basketball, hockey, jai-alai, lacrosse, soccer, race car driving). However, actual benefits for sports skills after octacosanol supplementation has not been documented.

VII. POLLEN

Use by athletes of bee or flower pollen has attracted a considerable amount of attention from the lay press.[794] Claims of ergogenic attributes of pollen have sprung from anecdotal testimonials or observations. Proponents claim pollen is a perfect food, although perusal of literature from pollen companies containing nutrient compositions reveal almost negligible amounts of vitamin B12, although other vitamins and minerals are present in small amounts, as well as the presence of protein, carbohydrates, and fats.

A study by Korchemny[794] reported improved recovery of pollen-supplemented track athletes from repeated races compared to controls. Pollen-extract tablets containing cernitins (plant growth factors — possibly sterols) were shown to increase work capacity of Polish weightlifters 70 to 120% compared to 30% for controls.[906] A study by Fjalkowski (cited by Steban[907]) on Polish weightlifters receiving cernitine-containing bee pollen tablets found significant decreases in lactate and improvements in EKG and respiratory parameters. A French allergen-free pollen extract was administered to malnourished patients, postsurgical patients, or geriatrics.[908] Very good results were seen for 67% of patients for weight gain, restoration of appetite, and reduction of debility. Urinary steroid excretion was significantly increased. Blood parameters, such as total protein, calcium, and phosphorus levels were normalized in supplemented groups, but not in control groups. Healing of bone fractures was accelerated. Doses ranged from 3 to 6 gelules per day for 8 d to 2 months, each gelule containing 6 mg of a lipid-soluble pollen extract and 20 mg of an aqueous pollen extract.

A product named Polbax® is produced from fertilized pollen tubes at a specific growth stage to provide measurable levels of superoxide dismutase (SOD) activity (1 g = 4 mcg CuZnSOD).[909] Antioxidant activity of Polbax® was confirmed in both *in vitro* and *in vivo* studies, with an increase of rabbit serum SOD activity after oral administration.[909] A study that did not specify methodological parameters, except for administration of Polbax® or placebo for 4 weeks, found significant reductions in post-exercise MDA levels in serum and muscle, significant reductions in lactate levels, and higher muscle glycogen levels after exercise attributed to the Polbax® group.[909] These results suggest that an antioxidant effect may have been apparent, but no further conclusions on ergogenic effects of Polbax® can be made until more experimental details are available.

However, four American studies and one British double-blind placebo study did not find ergogenic effects from bee pollen administration.[794,907,910–912] Collegiate swimmers were given ten tablets daily of bee pollen from an unspecified source.[907] Although significant improvements in serum potassium and hematocrit were seen after analysis by t-test, ANACOV statistical analysis found no significant differences. Performance was not different from the placebo group. Other blood parameters were unchanged. Eighteen high school cross-country runners received either four capsules of Cernelle Pollitabs, Cernelle pollen protein extract, or placebo capsules for 12 weeks.[910] Blood levels of potassium, hemoglobin, and hematocrits as well as 3-mile run times were not affected by the pollen or pollen protein supplementation. A 6-week course of supplementation with an unspecified amount of Pollitabs to 20 adolescent swimmers found no differences in strength, endurance, VO$_2$max, hemoglobin, or hematocrit levels between placebo (cod liver oil) and pollen groups.[911] However, the pollen group missed four total days of training from respiratory tract infections, while the placebo group lost 27 d. The authors suggested that a longer period of study may have found significant improvements in performance due to training time differences. A thesis cited by Williams[794] found no effects of 1350 or 2700 mg of bee pollen on the performance and recovery of repeated treadmill work tasks. Five trained endurance runners were studied for 3 weeks; 75 d of bee pollen supplementation (400 mg/d) did not affect VO$_2$max, forced vital capacity, forced expiration volume, grip strength, body fat, or body weight;[912] 46 normal subjects were employed in this double-blind study.

In summary, effects of bee pollen on human athletic performance are ambiguous. European studies find benefits, while American studies do not. While many forms of bee pollen are available, most studies used Pollitabs from one manufacturer. Further research to reproduce European findings on weightlifters are necessary. Dosage and length of administration are two variables not fully considered. Allergic reactions are possible and have been reported with pollen preparations, with anaphylactic shock a consideration.

Until further research confirms possible ergogenic effects of certain products, guidelines for dosages of pollen products as ergogenic aids would be premature.

VIII. SUCCINATES

Succinic acid is a component of the Krebs cycle, and as such is added to several dietary supplements with accompanying claims of ergogenesis.

Only one report of succinate on exercise performance was found.[913] Fasted male mice (serving as their own controls) were fed 0, 30, or 300 mg/kg sodium succinate, and swim tests to exhaustion started at 30, 60, and 120 min post-feeding. The only group to show improvement in swim times was the 300 mg/kg group 2 h after feeding (455 vs. 389 sec). Retesting of swim times 3 h after initial swim tests revealed no effects of succinate. Chronic feeding (7 d of 20 mg/ml succinate in drinking water) did not affect swim times. Results suggested that large doses of sodium succinate may improve exercise performance in swimming mice under certain conditions, and that extrapolation to humans would indicate that huge doses of succinate need to be studied for a possible ergogenic effect. No guidelines in humans for succinate supplementation exist at this time.

IX. COMMERCIALLY AVAILABLE SUBSTANCES WITH NO TESTING

Many reputed ergogenic aids are available to the public that have not been tested for effects on human physical performance. Literally hundreds of different combinations of nutrients and/or foodstuffs can be found in pharmacies, health food stores, muscle magazine advertisements, mail order catalogs, gyms, and even grocery stores. Most consist of "megadoses" of vitamins (usually not A or D), and minerals. Some also contain very small amounts of compounds with ergogenic properties previously mentioned in this book. Obviously, rigorous testing of each product is both unfeasible and unnecessary, as many can be seen to contain inadequate amounts of nutrients at recommended dose levels.

In addition, many compounds are available that have not been tested by academic researchers. A partial list of such compounds includes α-ketoacids, ascorbyl palmitate, ATP, various individual or mixtures of individual amino acids, betaine (commonly referred to as trimethylglycine or TMG), boron, carnosine, chlorophyll, cytochrome c, citrulline malate, colloidal silicates, dihydroepiandrostendione (DHEA), 6-keto-diosgenin, gamma hydroxybutyrate (GHB), glutathione, glandulars (dried raw animal organs), glycosaminoglycans, numerous herbs, lactate, lipoic acid (thioctic acid), NAD, pantetheine, pyruvate, plant sterols (e.g., β-sitosterol), various protein hydrolysates, sarcosine, somatomedins, vanadium salts, various citric acid cycle intermediates, and almost any metabolic intermediate compound found in the human body. Each has a theoretical rationale for use, regardless of relevance to reality.

Chapter 9

DESCRIPTION OF RESEARCH VARIABLES FOR ERGOGENIC AIDS STUDIES

Studies to ascertain the effects of nutritional ergogenic aids are wrought with difficulties. An understanding of the research variables involved is essential to analysis of studies and resulting conclusions.

I. HUMAN SUBJECT VARIABILITY

Table 1 lists most of the experimental variables encountered by researchers using human subjects. Controlling every variable with known limits of accuracy and precision is unfeasible. Although investigators endeavor to control as many variables as possible, contributions from unknown or uncontrolled variables are difficult to assess and may greatly alter results. An example is the caffeine habituation status for studies involving caffeine. Until the observation that caffeine-naive subjects, but not subjects regularly consuming caffeine, responded better to supplemental caffeine, conflicting results among several comparable studies could not be reconciled.

Thus, measurements of human performance are frequently associated with large variabilities. If variability within or between subjects is large, and measured differences are small, a real effect may be masked and may not reach statistical significance. Likewise, it is possible that a majority of subjects may show favorable responses but still be an insufficient number to achieve significance for the group. In a practical setting, any benefit may be significant for trained, competitive athletes. For example, a substance that improves performance by 1 or 2% may not show a statistically significant effect when tested. However, this improvement becomes of significance in practical settings such as timed events and races. An improvement in performance of 1 or 2% for time to run 5 km would result in 10 or 18 s off a time of 16 min. This amounts to a large difference for competitive athletes, and quite possibly a margin of victory.

Therefore, for a single experiment, findings of favorable or unfavorable results cannot be conclusive for determining the effects of a substance. Results should be interpreted according to the context of the design and proposed uses for the test compound before applicability to practical settings can be inferred.

II. PLACEBO EFFECTS

The Latin term "I will please" defines placebo. The placebo effect is the change in performance incurred by the change in mental state of a subject who expects a change from whatever he/she was administered. Both positive and negative placebo effects have been seen, although positive effects tend to predominate since subjects generally want to perform better.

TABLE 1
Research Variables in Human Exercise Studies

Subjects	Age
	Body composition
	Circadian or menstrual rhythms
	Clothing/equipment changes
	Gender
	Genetics (individual metabolic and kinesiologic variabilities)
	Illnesses (acute or chronic)
	Injuries
	Learning effects of measured tasks
	Mental effects (placebo, Hawthorne, motivation in positive or negative directions)
	Pharmaceutical use
	Training (conditioning) status
	Travel/time zone changes
Nutrient parameters	Bioavailability of nutrient(s)
	Concurrent and previous supplement usage
	Dosage
	Dosing schedule (acute, sub-acute, chronic)
	Form of nutrient
	Mode of administration (oral, intravenous)
	Placebo applicability
	Single or multiple nutrients
	Time of administration relative to exercise
Diet	Caloric intake
	Composition (% protein, fat, carbohydrates)
	Deficiencies and excesses
	History
	Hydration status
	Presence/absence of inhibiting/stimulating substances to test compound
	Self-selected or supplied by investigator
Study design	Control (open, field, single-blind, double-blind, crossover periods, etc.)
	Cost constraints
	Endpoints chosen for measurement
	Grouping of subjects
	Length of study period (acute or chronic)
	Measurement parameter choices
	Null hypothesis
	Number (n)
	Randomization
	Time-course of dosing, measurements
Measurement methods	Applicability to null hypothesis
	Assay characteristics (reproducibility, accuracy, precision, ease, cost)
	Equipment capabilities
	Objective or subjective
	Type of measurements (performance, physiological, biochemical)

TABLE 1 (continued)
Research Variables in Human Exercise Studies

Investigators	Competency
	Preconceived bias (positive or negative)
	Tone of report
Exercise	Type (aerobic or anaerobic)
	Duration
	Frequency
	Intensity (% VO$_2$max)
Results interpretation	Conclusion verified by results
	Publication goals
	Relevance of arbitrary level of significance to practical settings
	Speculation clearly listed as such
	Statistical analysis

The placebo effect is but one manifestation of the Hawthorne effect, which is a change in performance attributable to the subject's knowledge of simply being involved in a study, regardless of whether or not the subject received anything. Bias of results from expectations of the researcher is known as a halo effect. For these reasons, a study design called double-blind placebo-controlled has been accepted as the optimal design for studies of ergogenic aids. In these studies, neither the investigator nor the subject knows the identity of the test compound. Comparison of the placebo group to a control group receiving no aids will further strengthen the design.

Another factor to increase objectivity is to employ a crossover design, wherein a subject would get both a placebo and the active substance in a random, double-blind fashion. However, care must be taken to randomize when placebo or active agent is administered. Many studies with adequate experimental controls otherwise gave equivocal results because the placebo was administered first, and then the active agent administered second. This allows effects of training to continue during the study period, which would give improved performance to the second group and thus bias conclusions. The proper design would be to randomize which subject receives placebo or active agent first before crossover. These points are mentioned because many putative ergogenic aids have shown promising results when tested in uncontrolled situations or even what appeared to be well-controlled studies, but when subjected to more rigorous tests, most of these putative aids have shown no effect.

A classic illustration of the placebo effect is the recent report by Ariel.[914] A group of weightlifters were told by investigators that they would receive injections of anabolic steroids which would increase lean body mass. The subjects actually received injections of water, an inert placebo. Greater training gains were seen during the "placebo" period than a pre-placebo period, reaching significance in three of four exercises. The results approximated those expected for anabolic steroid administration, indicating the importance of controlling placebo effects.

III. APPLICABILITY OF ANIMAL RESEARCH

Animal research is important to determine safety, mechanisms of action, or biochemical processes that are difficult or unethical to determine in human subjects. However, the applicability to humans of results from animal studies is poorly understood owing to differences in physiology and methods of experimentation. A favorable result in animal studies may not be found in humans simply because experimental variables are more difficult to control for human subjects. Differences in muscle fiber types, training regimens, kinesiology, muscle mass, etc. may also confound comparisons. Regardless, animal research is less costly, free of placebo effects, and can answer basic hypotheses.

IV. SUFFICIENCY OF CURRENT RESEARCH

As is evident from this chapter and other thorough reviews of nutritional ergogenic aids,[8,33,34,199] a lack of research exists on the effects of many nutritional ergogenic aids, which has aided the credibility given to many unsubstantiated claims. This lack exists for several reasons. Relatively few groups (academic or corporate) are sufficiently funded to perform the rigorous, time-consuming, and expensive work required to explore effects of ergogenic aids fully. Sheer numbers of possible ergogenic aids and their combinations present a logistical nightmare for researchers. Human subjects are poor experimental models. Research showing no effects from low doses of a potential ergogenic aid discourages further research with higher doses. Dose-response studies are almost nonexistent. Companies with a particular product are reticent to fund at great expense a study that may have a negative impact on the marketability of that product when the company can support the product by locating academic research findings in the scientific literature indirectly related to the product. Academic researchers are more interested in elucidating mechanisms than being a product-testing facility. No central testing facility exists or is required for nutritional supplements or ergogenic aids. Companies selling nutritional supplements would rather compete among themselves than cooperate. Paradoxically, when nutrients are studied and shown to possess effects that are clinically useful, they are automatically categorized by law, not as nutrients but as drugs, if a claim of effectiveness is made. As such, a compound would become an Investigational New Drug, subject to a New Drug Application before claims could legally be made. Of course, the time (2 to 10 years) and cost (at least $2 million) of new drug approval prohibit both initial studies and applications to regulatory agencies. In addition, use patents are not generally given to nutrients, meaning that if someone proved, for example, that coenzyme Q_{10} was effective for improving exercise performance in patients recovering from cardiovascular disease and was granted approval to make these claims, anyone else could market coenzyme Q_{10} at a much reduced price, since no patent protection would be available. Thus, attainment of regulatory recognition for any nutritional ergogenic aid would amount to economic suicide. For this reason, there are no "approved" ergogenic aids by government regulatory agencies (Food and Drug Administration in the United States). This does not mean that there are no effective ergogenic aids.

Some obvious deficiencies in ergogenic aid research are apparent. First, the consideration of dose should be reiterated. For most nutrients, pharmacological data on normal subjects are available which can be used to choose an optimal dose and schedule to produce a desired response (e.g., peak serum concentration). Second, mixtures of several nutrients that affect one or related metabolic pathways have seldom been tested. The possibilities of synergistic combinations remain unexplored. Third, experimental designs to mimic popular exercises, such as weightlifting and "dance" aerobics to lower body fat levels are seldom encountered. When researchers more closely examine the exercises performed by many athletes and nonathletes, more popular credibility will be given to such research. Fourth, increasing collaboration between academic researchers and commercial interests may lead to benefits for each. Fifth, nutritional education in elementary, middle, and high schools is not stressed sufficiently. Ignorance of even basic nutritional knowledge leads to rampant proliferation of needless and useless products. Sixth, the legal framework regulating advertising claims and categorization of nutrients and drugs is becoming increasingly outdated, less applicable, and unenforceable.

V. NUTRITIONAL ERGOGENIC AIDS — FOODS OR DRUGS?

The previous discussion raises the issue of whether use of naturally-occurring compounds in doses far exceeding their potential intake from foodstuffs constitutes a pharmaceutical usage (which would be subject to rigorous and costly demonstration of safety and efficacy) or rather, an extreme example of food usage (which has almost no restrictions other than safety and lack of ability to make claims of efficacy). Therapeutic claims for any substance are only permitted for drugs (pharmaceuticals), which are defined as "...any component which is intended to furnish pharmacological activity or other direct effect in the diagnosis, cure, mitigation, treatment or prevention of disease, or to affect the structure or any function of the body of man or other animals."[9][15] By this definition, even water (when claimed to rehydrate the body after physical exertion or sweating) can legally be considered a drug and thus can be subject to determination of safety and efficacy. Obviously, enforcement of claims for foods is quite difficult in practice, with a large "gray area" that is almost unenforceable. Since exercise enhancement is not a life-threatening disease, enforcement of claims for nutrients affecting exercise is not pursued. Nevertheless, the entire field of nutritional ergogenic aids has acquired a "gray" flavor, hampering legitimate scientific inquiry of effects of nutrients on exercise performance. Naturally, many companies take advantage of this "gray" area and promote products via outlandish or unsubstantiated claims. Information and knowledge on effects of nutritional ergogenic aids from well-designed and well-conducted scientific studies in published, accessible formats offer a way to turn gray areas into black and white. Nutritional ergogenic aids are both foods and drugs.

Chapter 10

SUMMARY AND GUIDELINES FOR USE OF NUTRITIONAL ERGOGENIC AIDS

The field of ergogenic aids and human physical performance has reached a point where conclusive experiments can be performed to answer basic questions. One can speculate, with a large degree of certainty, that psychological and training effects on performance are much greater than physiological effects of ergogenic aids. However, in cases where training, motivation, and talent are already optimized, ergogenic aids may provide a small but significant improvement in performance. Also, in practical settings, nutritional ergogenic aids provide a placebo effect not attainable otherwise.

Perhaps the variable least controlled overall is dosage. As can be seen in Table 2 of Chapter 3, the only adequately controlled studies that show an ergogenic effect of B vitamins are those with the highest doses. Similarly, a dose-response for vitamin C, carnitine, ornithine, and caffeine is seen. Very few studies examined effects of more than one dose level of a given nutrient. Thresholds for ergogenic effects of nutrients have seldom been considered. Clearly, consideration of dose is required for future research on nutritional ergogenic acids.

Table 1 offers guidelines for use of those nutritional ergogenic aids for which available research has shown benefits for performance or for health conditions found in athletes. Table 1 illustrates the well-known advantages of water, electrolyte, and carbohydrate manipulations to maintain and enhance long-term endurance performance. Protein intake must be maintained within certain limits to prevent muscle mass loss. Bicarbonate loading for short-term, anaerobic work and caffeine ingestion for endurance events have shown sufficient ergogenic effects to be included for the population of exercising individuals as a whole, even though not everyone will benefit. Other nutrients (omega-3 fatty acids, B vitamins, minerals, certain amino acids, and antioxidants) have some data suggesting helpful properties, and they have been listed as speculative since confirmation of these properties is not as extensive as for water, electrolytes, carbohydrates, protein, bicarbonate, and caffeine. Doses chosen have shown safety in the reports cited in this book.

From the available data, it is evident that manipulation of dietary intake of particular nutrients may maintain and enhance certain aspects of exercise performance for a significant percentage of users. Many studies of nutrients have produced preliminary data that may develop into useful and safe ergogenic aids with further study. As nutrients in general are given more credence for their biological attributes, nutritional ergogenic aids will become more sophisticated and effective. Hopefully, pertinent research will be increased in order to define efficacy or lack thereof for nutritional ergogenic aids.

TABLE 1
Guidelines for Use of Nutritional Aids with Documented Ergogenic Effects

Nutrient	Subject/exercise type	Guidelines
Water and electrolytes:	Trained and untrained endurance events lasting >1 5 h and high sweat loss activities	400–600 ml 15–20 min before event, followed by 100–200 ml every 2–3 km 15 min (see Carbohydrate replenishment)
Carbohydrates:		
Pre-exercise meal	Trained and untrained/ any event or practice	3–4 h before event eat ≥300 g carbohydrates, low fat, low fiber
Carbohydrate loading	Trained/single event lasting >1.5 h	Eat 60–79% of calories from carbohydrates (500–600 g daily); start 1 week before event; taper exercise load down by 1/2 every 2nd day until event
Carbohydrate replenishment	Trained and untrained/ endurance events lasting >1.5 h	Consume 1–1.5 cups of sports drink every 15–20 min during event
Glycogen resynthesis	Trained and untrained/ any exhaustive exercise and for daily strenuous events	Start carbohydrate (sugars) intake immediately after exercise; 0.7 g glucose/kg body weight (500–700 g total in 24 h) as sports drinks and foods
Protein:	Untrained/ weightlifting or long endurance events	100–200 g protein daily (2–2.5 g protein/kg/d); consume adequate calories; lean foods or protein powders
Omega-3 fatty acids (speculative):	Untrained and trained/ endurance and strength training	2–4 g daily of omega-3 fatty acids GLA, ALA, EPA, DHA) for long-term periods; food sources: salmon, mackerel, sardines, herrings, fish oil supplements, flaxseed oil
B vitamins (speculative):	Untrained and trained/ endurance training	100–1000 mg thiamine/d 100–2000 mg pantothenate/d
	Fine motor control events (shooting, skill sports)	Short-term only: 300 mg thiamine/d; 300 mg pyridoxine/d; 600 mcg B_{12}/d
Antioxidant nutrients (speculative):	Untrained and trained/ and endurance exercise (prevent cell damage and enhance recovery)	Long-term daily doeses: β-carotene: 25,000–100,000 IU Vitamin E (d-α-tocopherols): 400–800 IU Vitamin C: 1000–2000 mg Selenium: 100–200 mcg (selenite)
Sodium bicarbonate:	Trained/ exhaustive anaerobic events lasting 1–7 min and repeated	0.2–0.3 g/kg body weight 1–3 h before exercise with water
Calcium:	Untrained and trained/ thin, amenorrheic women and osteoporosis	500–1500 mg calcium daily as calcium citrate or calcium citrate/malate
Iron:	Untrained and trained/ anemic subjects (endurance events)	15–50 mg iron daily from organic chelates (fumarate, gluconate, glycinate, etc.)
Caffeine:	Trained, caffeine-naive/ endurance events	200–300 mg (2–3 cups brewed coffee) 1 h before event

REFERENCES

1. **Read, M. H. and McGuffin, S. L.**, The effect of B-complex supplementation on endurance performance, *J. Sports Med.*, 23, 178, 1983

2. **Lamb, D. R., Ed.,** *Physiology of Exercise: Responses and Adaptations*, Macmillan, New York, 1978, 355

3. **Brooks G. A. and Fahey, T. D., Eds.,** Ergogenic aids, in *Exercise Physiology: Human Bioenergetics and its Application,* John Wiley & Sons, New York, 1984, 611

4. **deVries, H. A., Ed.,** Special aids to performance, in *Physiology of Exercise for Physical Education and Athletics,* 3rd ed., W.C Brown, Dubuque, IA, 1980, 533.

5. **Karpovich, P. V., Ed.,** Ergogenic aids in work and sports, in *Physiology of Muscular Activity,* 6th ed., W S Saunders, Philadelphia, 1965, 261

6. **McArdle, W. D., Katch, E. L, and Katch, V. L., Eds.,** Special aids to performance and conditioning, in *Exercise Physiology Energy, Nutrition, and Human Performance,* 2nd ed., Lea & Febiger, Philadelphia, 1986, 401

7. **Morgan, W. P., Ed.,** *Ergogenic Aids and Muscular Performance,* Academic Press, New York, 1972

8. **Williams, M. H., Ed.,** *Ergogenic Aids in Sports,* Human Kinetics Publishers, Champaign, IL, 1983

9. **Williams, M. H., Ed.,** *Drugs and Athletic Performance,* Charles C Thomas, Springfield, IL, 1974.

10. **Macintyre, J. G.,** Growth hormone and athletes. *Sports Med.*, 4, 129, 1987.

11. **Wagner, J. C.,** Enhancement of athletic performance with drugs An overview *Sports Med.*, 12(4), 250, 1991.

12. **Committee on Substance Abuse Research and Education,** *USOC/IOC Banned Drugs,* U.S Olympic Committee, Colorado Springs, CO, 1986

13. **Goldman, B.,** *Death in the Locker Room,* Icarus Press, South Bend, IN, 1984.

14. **Haupt, H. A.,** Drugs in athletics. *Clin Sports Med.*, 8, 561, 1989

15. **Haupt, H A. and Rovere, G. D.,** Anabolic steroids: a review of the literature, *Am J Sports Med.*, 12, 469, 1984.

16. **Hickson, R. C., Ball, K. L., and Falduto, M. T.,** Adverse effects of anabolic steroids, *Med Toxicol Adverse Drug Exp.*, 4, 254, 1989.

17. **Kochakian, C. D., Ed.,** *Anabolic-Androgenic Steroids,* Springer-Verlag, New York, 1976

18. **Kibble, M. W. and Ross, M. B.,** Adverse effects of anabolic steroids in athletes, *Clin Pharm.*, 6, 686, 1987

19. **Kleiner, S. M.,** Performance-enhancing aids in sport: health consequences and nutritional alternatives, *J Am Coll Nutr.*, 10(2), 115, 1991

20. **Kruskemper, H. L., Ed.,** *Anabolic Steroids,* Academic Press, New York, 1968

21. **Wright, J. E.,** Anabolic steroids and athletes, *Exer Sport Sci Rev.*, 8, 149, 1980

22. **Wright, J. E. and Stone, M. H.,** *Anabolic Drug Use by Athletes Literature Review,* National Strength and Conditioning Association, Lincoln, NE, 1985

23. **Alen, M. and Rahkila, P.,** Reduced high-density lipoprotein-cholesterol in power athletes: use of male sex hormone derivatives, an atherogenic factor, *Int J Sports Med.*, 5, 341, 1984

24. **Alen, M., Rahkila, P., and Marniemi, J.,** Serum lipids in power athletes self-administering testosterone and anabolic steroids, *Int J Sports Med.*, 6, 139, 1985

25. **Hurley, B. F., Seals, D. R., Hagberg, J. M., Goldberg, A. C., Ostrove, S. M., Holloszy, J. O., Wiest, W. G., and Goldberg, A. P.,** High-density cholesterol in bodybuilders and powerlifters, *JAMA,* 252, 507, 1984

26. **Kantor, M. A., Bianchini, A., Bernier, D., Sady, S. P., and Thompson, P. D.,** Androgens reduce HDL_2-cholesterol and increase hepatic triglyceride lipase activity, *Med Sci Sports Exer.*, 17, 462, 1985

27. **Webb, O. L., Laskarzewski, P. M., and Glueck, C. J.,** Severe depression of high-density lipoprotein cholesterol levels in weight lifters and body builders by self-administered exogenous testosterone and anabolic-androgenic steroids, *Metabolism,* 33, 971, 1984.

28 McKillop, G. and Ballantyne, D., Lipoprotein analysis in bodybuilders, *Int J Cardiol* , 17, 281, 1987

29. Kleiner, S. M., Calabrese, L. H., Fielder, K. M., Naito, H. K., and Skibinski, C. I., Dietary influences on cardiovascular disease risk in anabolic steroid using and non-using bodybuilders, *J Am Coll Nutr* , 8, 109, 1989

30 Haskell, W., Scala, J., and Whittam, J., Eds., *Nutrition and Athletic Performance*, Bull Publishing, Palo Alto, CA, 1982

31. Fox, E. L., Ed., *Ross Symposium on Nutrient Utilization During Exercise*, Ross Laboratories, Columbus, OH, 1983.

32 Knuttgen, H. G., Vogel, J. A., and Poortmans, J., Eds., *Biochemistry of Exercise*, Human Kinetics Publishers, Champaign, IL, 1983.

33 Williams, M. H., Ed., *Nutritional Aspects of Human Physical and Athletic Performance*, 2nd ed , Charles C Thomas, Springfield, IL, 1985.

34 Bucci, L.R., Nutritional ergogenic aids, in *Nutrition in Exercise and Sport*, Hickson, J. F and Wolinsky, I , Eds , CRC Press, Boca Raton, FL, 1989, 107.

35. Lemon, P. W. R. and Proctor, D. N., Protein intake and athletic performance, *Sports Med* , 12(5), 313, 1991.

36. Maughan, R. J. and Noakes, T. D., Fluid replacement and exercise stress A brief review of studies on fluid replacement and some guidelines for the athlete, *Sports Med* , 12(1), 16, 1991.

37. Costill, D. L. and Hargreaves, M., Carbohydrate nutrition and fatigue, *Sports Med* , 13(2), 86, 1992.

38. Greenleaf, J. E., The body's need for fluids, in *Nutrition and Athletic Performance*, Haskell, W , Scala, J., and Whittam, J., Eds., Bull Publishing, Palo Alto, CA, 1982

39 Herbert, W. G., Water and electrolytes, in *Ergogenic Aids in Sports*, Williams, M. H , Ed , Human Kinetics Publishers, Champaign, IL, 1983, 56.

40. Williams, M. H., Ed., The role of water and electrolytes in physical activity, in *Nutritional Aspects of Human Physical and Athletic Performance*, 2nd ed., Charles C Thomas, Springfield, IL, 1985, 219

41. Pivarnik, J. M., Water and electrolytes during exercise, in *Nutrition in Exercise and Sport*, Hickson, J. F. and Wolinsky, I., Eds , CRC Press, Boca Raton, FL, 1989, 185.

42. Gisolfi, C. V., Water and electrolyte metabolism in exercise, in *Ross Symposium on Nutrient Utilization During Exercise*, Fox, E. L., Ed., Ross Laboratories, Columbus, OH, 1983, 21.

43. Fink, W. J., Fluid intake for maximizing athletic performance, in *Nutrition and Athletic Performance*, Haskell, W., Scala, J., and Whittam, J., Eds., Bull Publishing, Palo Alto, CA, 1982, 52.

44 Greenhaff, P. L. and Clough, P. J., Predictors of sweat loss in man during prolonged exercise, *Eur J Appl Physiol* , 58, 348, 1989.

45 American College of Sports Medicine, Position stand on prevention of thermal injuries during distance running, *Med Sci Sports Exer.*, 16, ix, 1984

46. Deschamps, A., Levy, R. D., Cosio, M. G., Marliss, E. B., and Magder, S., Effect of saline infusion on body temperature and endurance during heavy exercise, *J Appl Physiol* , 66, 2799, 1989.

47. Noakes, T. D., Goodwin, N., Rayner, B. L., Branken, T., and Taylor, R. K. N., Water intoxication: a possible complication during endurance exercise, *Med Sci Sports Exer* , 17, 370, 1985

48 Buskirk, E. R. and Puhl, S., Nutritional beverages: exercise and sport, in *Nutrition in Exercise and Sport*, Hickson, J F and Wolinsky, I , Eds., CRC Press, Boca Raton, FL, 1989, 201

49 Miller, G. D. and Massaro, E. J., Carbohydrate in ultra-endurance performance, in *Nutrition in Exercise and Sport*, Hickson, J. F and Wolinsky, I., Eds., CRC Press, Boca Raton, FL, 1989, 51

50. **Pate, T. D. and Brunn, J. C.,** Fundamentals of carbohydrate metabolism, in *Nutrition in Exercise and Sport*, Hickson, J. F and Wolinsky, I., Eds., CRC Press, Boca Raton, FL, 1989, 37

51 **Valeriani, A.,** The need for carbohydrate intake during endurance exercise, *Sports Med*, 12(6), 349, 1991.

52. **Nagle, F. J. and Bassett, D. R.,** Energy metabolism, in *Nutrition in Exercise and Sport*, Hickson, J F and Wolinsky, I., Eds., CRC Press, Boca Raton, FL, 1989, 87

53 **Friedman, J. E., Neufer, P. D., and Dohm, G. L.,** Regulation of glycogen resynthesis following exercise. Dietary considerations, *Sports Med.*, 11(4), 232, 1991.

54 **Williams, M. H., Ed.,** The role of carbohydrates in physical activity, in *Nutritional Aspects of Human Physical and Athletic Performance*, 2nd ed., Charles C Thomas, Springfield, IL, 1985, 58

55 **Sherman, W. H.,** Carbohydrates, muscle glycogen and muscle glycogen supercompensation, in *Ergogenic Aids in Sports*, Williams, M. H , Ed., Human Kinetics Publishers, Champaign, IL, 1983, 3

56 **Christensen, E. H. and Hansen, O.,** Respiratorischer Quotient und O_2-Aufnahme, *Scand Arch Physiol*, 81, 180, 1939.

57 **Ahlborg, B. G., Bergstrom, J., Brohult, J., Ekelund, L. G., Hultman, E., and Maschio, G.,** Human muscle glycogen content and capacity for prolonged exercise after different diets, *Foersvarsmedicin*, 3, 85, 1967

58 **Bergstrom, J., Hermansen, L., Hultman, E., and Saltin, B.,** Diet, muscle glycogen, and physical performance, *Acta Physiol Scand*, 71, 140, 1967

59 **Gollnick, P. D., Pernow, B., Essen, B., Jansson, E., and Saltin, B.,** Availability of glycogen and plasma FFA for substrate utilization in leg muscle of man during exercise, *Clin Physiol*, 1, 1, 1980

60 **Karlsson, J. and Saltin, B.,** Diet, muscle glycogen and exercise performance, *J Appl Physiol*, 31, 203, 1971 .

61 **Slovic, P.,** What helps the long distance runner run?, *Nutr Today*, 10, 18, 1975.

62 **Scully, B.,** Effects of variation in diet and intensity of exercise on blood lactate levels and performance time, *Int Congr Phys. Act Sci.*, (Abstr.) CISAP, Quebec City, 1976

63 **Martin, B., Robinson, S., and Robertshaw, D.,** Influence of diet on leg uptake of glucose during heavy exercise, *Am J Clin Nutr*, 31, 62, 1978.

64 **Goforth, H., Hodgdon, J. A., and Hilderbrand, R. L.,** A double-blind study of the effects of carbohydrate loading upon endurance performance, *Med Sci Sports Exer*, 12, 108, 1980.

65 **Maughan, R. and Poole, D.,** The effects of a glycogen-loading regimen on the capacity to perform anaerobic exercise, *Eur J Appl Physiol.*, 46, 211, 1981.

66 **Durnin, J.,** Muscle in sports medicine — nutrition and muscular performances, *Int J Sports Med*, Suppl 1, 52, 1982.

67 **Siemann, A.,** S-T segment changes during monitored bicycle ergometer exertion following varied carbohydrate feeding and vitamin B6 supplementation, *1983 AAHPERD Convention*, Research Papers (Abstr.), AAHPERD, Reston, VA, 1983

68 **Piehl, K.,** Time course for refilling of glycogen stores in human muscle fibers following exercise-induced glycogen depletion, *Acta Physiol Scand*, 90, 297, 1974

69 **Wilmore, J. H. and Freund, B. J.,** Nutritional enhancement of athletic performance, in *Nutrition and Exercise*, Winick, M., Ed., John Wiley & Sons, New York, 1986, 67

70 **Saltin, B. and Hermansen, L.,** Glycogen stores and prolonged severe exercise, in *Nutrition and Physical Activity*, Blix, G , Ed , Almqvist & Wiksells, Uppsala, Sweden, 1967

71 **Astrand, P. O.,** Diet and athletic performance, *Fed Proc*, 26, 1772, 1967

72 **Bergstrom, J. and Hultman, E.,** Muscle glycogen synthesis after exercise: an enhancing factor localized to muscle cells in man, *Nature*, 210(5033), 309, 1966

73 **Hermansen, L., Hultman, E., and Saltin, B.,** Muscle glycogen during prolonged severe exercise, *Acta Physiol Scand*, 71, 129, 1967

74 Tremblay, A. and Allard, C., Nutrition and physical activity *Union Med Can* , 109, 636, 1980

75 Sherman, W. M., Costill, D. L., Fink, W. J., and Miller, J. M., The effect of exercise and diet manipulation on muscle glycogen and its subsequent utilization during performance, *Int J Sports Med* , 2, 114, 1981.

76 Sherman, W. M., Costill, D. L., Fink, W., and Miller, J., Carbohydrate loading: a practical approach, *Med Sci Sports Exer* , 13, 90, 1981

77. Sherman, W. and Costill, D., The marathon: dietary manipulation to optimize performance, *Am J Sports Med* , 12(1), 44, 1984.

78 Greenhaff, P. L., Gleeson, M., and Maughan, R. J., The effects of dietary manipulation on blood acid-base status and the performance of high intensity exercise, *Eur J Appl Physiol.*, 56, 331, 1987.

79 Wooton, S. A. and Williams, C., Influence of carbohydrate status on performance during maximal exercise, *Int J Sports Med* , 5, S126, 1984.

80 Costill, D. L., Carbohydrates for exercise: dietary demands for optimal performance, *Int J Sports Med* , 9, 1, 1988.

81 Sherman, W. M. and Wimer, G. S., Insufficient dietary carbohydrate during training: does it impair athletic performance?, *Int J Sport Nutr* , 1, 28, 1991

82 Coyle, E. F., Effects of glucose polymers feedings on fatigability and the metabolic response to prolonged strenuous exercise, in *Ross Symposium on Nutrient Utilization During Exercise*, Fox, E L., Ed , Ross Laboratories, Columbus, OH, 1983, 43

83 Ivy, J. L., Miller, W., Dover, V., Goodyear, L. G., Sherman, W. M., and Farrell, S., Enhanced performance with carbohydrate supplements during endurance exercise, in *Ross Symposium on Nutrient Utilization During Exercise*, Fox, E. L., Ed , Ross Laboratories, Columbus, OH, 1983, 54.

84 Costill, D. L., Sherman, W. M., Fink, W. J., Maresh, C., Witten, M., and Miller, J. M., The role of dietary carbohydrate in muscle glycogen resynthesis after strenuous running, *Am J Clin Nutr* , 34, 1831, 1981.

85 Coyle, E. F., Coggan, A. R., Hemmert, M. K., Lowe, R. C., and Walters, T. J., Substrate usage during prolonged exercise following a pre-exercise meal, *J Appl Physiol* , 59, 429, 1985.

86 Neufer, P. D., Costill, D. L., Flynn, M. G., Kirwan, J. P., and Mitchell, J. B., Improvements in exercise performance: effects of carbohydrate feedings and diet, *J Appl Physiol* , 62, 983, 1987

87 Costill, D. L. and Miller, J., Nutrition for endurance sport: carbohydrate and fluid balance, *Int J Sports Med* , 1, 2, 1980.

88. Sherman, W. M., Brodowicz, G., Wright, D. A., Allen, W. K., and Simonsen, J., Effects of 4h pre-exercise carbohydrate feedings on cycling performance, *Med Sci Sports Exer* , 21, 598, 1989

89. Wright, D. A. and Sherman, W. M., Carbohydrate feedings 3 h before and during exercise improve cycling performance, *Med Sci Sports Exer* , 21, S58, 1989

90 Fruth, J. M. and Gisolfi, C. V., Effects of carbohydrate consumption on endurance performance: fructose versus glucose, in *Ross Symposium on Nutrient Utilization During Exercise*, Fox, E. L., Ed., Ross Laboratories, Columbus, OH, 1983, 68

91. Langenfeld, M. E., Utilization of glucose polymers in endurance bicycle racing, in *Ross Symposium on Nutrient Utilization During Exercise*, Fox, E L , Ed., Ross Laboratories, Columbus, OH, 1983, 60

92. Cade, R., Spooner, G., Schlein, E., Pickering, M., and Dean, R., Effect of fluid, electrolyte and glucose replacement during exercise on performance, body temperature, rate of sweat loss, and compositional changes of extracellular fluid, *J Sports Med Phys Fit* , 12, 150, 1972

93. Ivy, J. L., Costill, D. L., Fink, W. J., and Lower, R. W., Influence of caffeine and carbohydrate feedings on endurance performance, *Med. Sci Sports Exer* , 11, 6, 1979

94 Coyle, E. F., Hagberg, J. M., Hurley, B. F., Martin, W. H., Ehsani, A. A., and Holloszy, J. O., Carbohydrate feeding during prolonged strenuous exercise can delay fatigue, *J Appl Physiol*, 55, 230, 1983.

95 Ivy, J. L., Miller, W., Dover, V., Goodyear, L. G., Sherman, W. M., Farrell, S., and Williams, H., Endurance improved by ingestion of a glucose polymer supplement, *Med Sci Sports Exer*, 15, 466, 1983

96 Macareg, P. V. J., Influence of carbohydrate-electrolyte ingestion on running endurance, in *Ross Symposium on Nutrient Utilization During Exercise*, Fox, E L , Ed., Ross Laboratories, Columbus, OH, 1983, 91

97 Bjorkman, O., Sahlin, K., Hagenfeldt, L., and Wahren, J., Influence of fructose and glucose ingestion on the capacity for long-term exercise in well-trained men, *Clin Physiol*, 4, 483, 1984

98 Coyle, E. F. and Coggan, A. R., Effectiveness of carbohydrate feeding in delaying fatigue during prolonged exercise, *Sports Med*, 1, 446, 1984

99 Hargreaves, M., Costill, D. L., Coggan, A., Fink, W. J., and Nishibata, I., Effect of carbohydrate feedings on muscle glycogen utilization and exercise performance, *Med Sci Sports Exer*, 16, 219, 1984

100 Costill, D. L., Carbohydrate nutrition before, during, and after exercise, *Fed Proc*, 44, 364, 1985

101 Askew, E. W., Claybaugh, J. R., Hashiro, G. M., Stokes, W. S., and Cucinell, S. A., Carbohydrate supplementation during exercise at high altitude, *Fed Proc*, 45, 972, 1986.

102 Coyle, E. F., Coggan, A. R., Hemmert, M. K., and Ivy, J. L., Muscle glycogen utilization during prolonged strenuous exercise when fed carbohydrate, *J Appl Physiol*, 61, 165, 1986

103 Foster, C., Thompson, N. M., Dean, J., and Kirkendall, D. T., Carbohydrate supplementation and performance in soccer players, *Med Sci Sports Exer*, 18, 012, 1986

104 Coggan, A. R and Coyle, E. F., Reversal of fatigue during prolonged exercise by carbohydrate infusion or ingestion, *J Appl Physiol*, 63, 2388, 1987

105 Sasaki, H., Maeda, J., Usui, S., and Ishiko, T., Effect of sucrose and caffeine ingestion on performance of prolonged strenuous exercise, *Int J Sports Med*, 8, 261, 1987

106. Seifert, J. G., Langenfeld, M. E., and Rudge, S. J., Effects of glucose polymer ingestion on ultraendurance bicycling performance, *Med Sci Sports Exer*, 18, S5, 1986.

107 Shephard, R. J. and Leatt, P., Carbohydrate and fluid needs of the soccer player, *Sports Med*, 4, 164, 1987.

108 Coggan, A. R. and Coyle, E. F., Effect of carbohydrate feedings during high-intensity exercise, *J Appl Physiol*, 65, 1703, 1988

109 Johnson, H. L., Nelson, R. A., and Consolazio, C. F., Effects of electrolyte and nutrient solutions on performance and metabolic balance, *Med Sci Sports Exer*, 20, 26, 1988

110 McLaren, D. and Otter, M., The effect of glucose and medium chain triglyceride ingestion on exercise metabolism, *J Sports Sci*, 6, 167, 1988.

111 Millard-Stafford, M. L., Cureton, K. J., and Ray, C. A., Effect of glucose polymer diet supplement on responses to prolonged successive swimming, cycling, and running, *Eur J Appl Physiol*, 58, 327, 1988.

112 Mitchell, J. B., Costill, D. L., Houmard, J. A., Flynn, M. G., and Fink, W. J., Effects of carbohydrate ingestion on gastric emptying and exercise performance, *Med Sci Sports Exer*, 20, 110, 1988

113 Mitchell, J. B., Costill, D. L., Houmard, J. A., Fink, W. J., and Pascoe, D. D., Influence of carbohydrate dosage on exercise performance and glycogen metabolism, *J Appl Physiol*, 67, 1843, 1989

114 Mouton, A. and Ribière, C., Conseils diététique pour un coureur de marathon, *Cah Nutr Diét*, 23, 75, 1988

115 Coggan, A. R. and Coyle, E. F., Metabolism and performance following carbohydrate ingestion late in exercise, *Med Sci Sports Exer*, 21, 59, 1989

116. **Murray, R., Paul, G. L., Seifert, J. G., Eddy, D. E., and Halaby, G. A.,** The effects of glucose, fructose, and sucrose ingestion during exercise, *Med. Sci Sports Exer ,* 21, 275, 1989

117. **Wheeler, K. B.,** Sports nutrition for the primary care physician: the importance of carbohydrate, *Phys Sportsmed ,* 17(5), 106, 1989

118. **Macdougal, J. D., Ward, G. R., Sale, D. G., and Sutton, J. R.,** Muscle glycogen repletion after high-intensity intermittent exercise. *J Appl. Physiol ,* 42, 129, 1977.

119. **Ivy, J. L., Katz, A. L., Cutler, C. L., Sherman, W. M., and Coyle, E. F.,** Muscle glycogen synthesis after exercise: effect of time of carbohydrate ingestion, *Am Physiol Soc.,* 64, 1480, 1988.

120. **Ivy, J. L., Lee, M. C., Brozinick, J. T., Jr., and Reed, M. J.,** Muscle glycogen storage after different amounts of carbohydrate ingestion, *J. Appl Physiol ,* 65(5), 2018, 1988.

121. **Blom, P. C. S., Vollestad, N. K., and Cotill, D. L.,** Factors affecting changes in muscle glycogen concentration during and after prolonged exercise, *Acta Physiol Scand ,* 128 (S556), 67, 1986

122. **Blom, P. C. S., Hostmark, A. T., Vaage, O., Kardel, K. R., and Maehlum, S.,** Effect of different post-exercise sugar diets on the rate of muscle glycogen synthesis, *Med Sci Sports Exer ,* 19, 491, 1987.

123 **Keizer, H. A., Kuipers, H., van Kranenburg, G., and Guerten, P.,** Influence of liquid and solid meals on muscle glycogen resynthesis, plasma fuel hormone response, and maximal physical working capacity, *Int. J Sports Med.,* 8, 99, 1986.

124. **Bergstrom, J. and Hultman, E.,** Synthesis of muscle glycogen in man after glucose and fructose infusion, *Acta Med Scand.,* 182, 93, 1967.

125. **Conlee, R. K., Lawler, R., and Ross, P.,** Effect of fructose or glucose ingestion on glycogen repletion in muscle and liver after exercise or fasting, *Med Sci Sports Exer ,* 14, 137, 1982

126. **Kiens, B., Raber, A. B., Valeur, A.-K., and Richter, E. A.,** Benefit of dietary simple carbohydrates on the early postexercise muscle glycogen repletion in male athletes, *Med Sci Sports Exer.,* 22, S88, 1990

127 **Costill, D. L., Pascoe, D. D., Fink, W. J., Robergs, R. A., and Barr, S. I.,** Impaired muscle glycogen resynthesis after eccentric exercise, *J Appl Physiol ,* 69, 46, 1990

128. **Sherman, W., Costill, D., Fink, W., Hagerman, F., and Armstrong, L.,** Effect of a 42 2km footrace and subsequent rest or exercise on muscle glycogen and enzymes, *J Appl Physiol ,* 55, 1219, 1983.

129. **O'Reilly, K. P., Warhol, M. J., Fielding, R. A., Frontera, W. R., and Meredith, C. N.,** Eccentric exercise-induced muscle damage impairs muscle glycogen repletion, *J Appl Physiol ,* 63, 252, 1987

130 **Myers, J., Atwood, J. E., Forbes, S., Evans, B., and Froelicher, V.,** Effect of fructose 1,6-diphosphate on exercise capacity in patients with peripheral vascular disease, *Int J Sports Med ,* 11(4), 259, 1990.

131. **Webb, W. R.,** Metabolic effects of fructose diphosphate in hypoxic and ischemic states, *J Thorac Cardiovasc Surg.,* 88, 863, 1984

132 **Lemon, P. W. R.,** Protein and exercise: update 1987, *Med Sci Sports Exer ,* 19, S179, 1987

133 **Kaufmann, D. A.,** Protein as an energy substrate during intense exercise, *Ann Sports Med ,* 5, 142, 1990.

134 **Dohm, G. L.,** Protein nutrition for the athlete, *Clin Sports Med ,* 3, 595, 1985

135 **Williams, M. H., Ed.,** The role of protein in physical exercise, in *Nutritional Aspects of Human Physical and Athletic Performance,* 2nd ed., Charles C Thomas, Springfield, IL, 1985, 120

136 **Consolazio, C. F., Johnson, H. L., Nelson, R. A., Dramise, J. G., and Skala, J. H.,** Protein metabolism during intensive physical training in the young adult, *Am J Clin Nutr ,* 28, 29, 1975.

137. **Astrand, P. and Rodahl, K., Eds.,** *Textbook of Work Physiology,* McGraw-Hill, New York, 1970.
138. **Kraut, H. and Müller, E. A.,** Muskelkrafte und Eiweissration, *Biochem Z* , 320, 302, 1950
139. **Kraut, H., Müller, E. A., and Müller-Wecker, H.,** Der Einfluss zu Zusammensetzung des Nahrungseiweisses auf Stickstoffbilanz und Muskeltraining, *Int Z Angew Physiol* , 17, 378, 1958
140. **Travers, P. and Campbell, W.,** The organism and speed and power, in *Fitness, Health and Work Capacity,* Larson, L , Ed , Macmillan, New York, 1974
141 **Rasch, P. and Pierson, W.,** The effect of a protein dietary supplement on muscular strength and hypertrophy, *Am J Clin Nutr.,* 11, 530, 1962.
142 **Rasch, P., Hamby, J. W., and Burns, H. J.,** Protein dietary supplementation and physical performance, *Med Sci Sports,* 1, 195, 1969.
143 **Oddoye, E. B. and Margen, S.,** Nitrogen balance studies in humans: long-term effect of high nitrogen intake on nitrogen accretion, *J Nutr* , 109, 363, 1979.
144 **Marable, N. L., Hickson, J. F., Korslund, M. K., Herbert, W. G., and Desjardins, R. F.,** Urinary nitrogen excretion as influenced by a muscle-building exercise program and protein intake variation, *Nutr Rep Int* , 19, 795, 1979
145 **Dragan, G. I., Vasiliu, A., and Georgescu, E.,** Effects of increased supply of protein on elite weight lifters, in *Milk Proteins '84,* Galesloot, T. E. and Timbergen, B. J., Eds , Pudoc, Waningen, Netherlands, 1985.
146 **Hecker, A. L. and Wheeler, K. B.,** Protein: a misunderstood nutrient for the athlete, *NSCA J* , 7(6), 28, 1985
147 **Frontera, W. R., Meredith, C. N., O'Reilly, K. P., Knuttgen, G., and Evans, W. J.,** Strength conditioning in older men: skeletal muscle hypertrophy and improved function, *J Appl Physiol.,* 64, 1038, 1988
148 **Stegink, L. D.,** Peptides in parenteral nutrition, in *Clinical Nutrition Update Amino Acids,* Greene, H L., Holliday, M A., and Munro, H M , Eds , AMA, Chicago, 1977, 192.
149 **Belikov, V. M. and Babayan, T. L.,** Mixtures of amino acids in human nutrition, *Russ Chem Rev.,* 40, 441, 1971
150 **Greene, H. L., Holliday, M. A., and Munro, H. M., Eds.,** *Clinical Nutrition Update,* AMA, Chicago, 1977.
151 **Blackburn, C. L., Grant, J. P., and Young, V. R., Eds.,** *Amino Acids Metabolism and Medical Applications,* John Wright, Boston, 1983
152 **Winitz, M., Seedman, D. A., and Graff, J.,** Studies in metabolic nutrition employing chemically defined diets. 1 Extended feeding of normal human adult males, *Am J Clin Nutr* , 23, 525, 1970
153 **Lowry, S. F., Legaspi, A., Albert, J. D., Horowitz, G. D., and Tracey, K. J.,** Thermogenic and nitrogen response to submaximal exercise in parenterally repleted normal man, *Am J Clin Nutr* , 46, 237, 1987.
154 **Hickson, J. F. and Wolinsky, I.,** Human protein intake and metabolism in exercise and sport, in *Nutrition in Exercise and Sport,* Hickson, J. F and Wolinsky, I., Eds , CRC Press, Boca Raton, FL, 1989, 5
155 **Wilkens, K. G.,** Nutritional care in diseases of the kidney, in *Food, Nutrition, and Diet Therapy,* Krause, M. V. and Mahan, L. K., Eds , W. B. Saunders, Philadelphia, 1984, 600
156 **Zaragoza, R., Renau-Piqueras, J., Portoles, M., Hernandez-Yago, J., and Jorda, A.,** Rats fed prolonged high protein diets show an increase in nitrogen metabolism and liver megamitochondria, *Arch Biochem Biophys* , 258, 426, 1987.
157 **Williams, M. H.,** The role of fat in physical activity, in *Nutritional Aspects of Human Physical and Athletic Performance,* 2nd ed., Charles C Thomas, Springfield, IL, 1985, 106
158. **Marcus, A. J.,** The eicosanoids in biology and medicine, *J Lipid Res* , 25, 1511, 1984
159 **Simopoulos, A. P.,** Omega-3 fatty acids in health and disease and in growth and development, *Am J Clin. Nutr* , 54, 438, 1991.

160   Nordoy, A., Is there a rational use for n-3 fatty acids (fish oils) in clinical medicine? *Drugs,* 42(3), 331, 1991

161   Schofield, G., Prostaglandin E₁ and the release of growth hormone in vitro, *Nature,* 228, 179, 1970.

162.   Hertelendy, F., Todd, H., Ehrhart, K., and Blute, R., Studies on growth hormone secretion. IV In vivo effects of prostaglandin E₁, *Prostaglandins,* 2, 79, 1972.

163.   Hertelendy, F., Studies on growth hormone secretion. VI. Effects of dibutyryl cyclic AMP, prostaglandin E₁, and indomethacin on growth hormone secretion, *Prostaglandins,* 6, 217, 1974.

164.   McKeown, B. A., John, T. M., and George, J. C., The effect of prostaglandin E₁ on plasma growth hormone, free fatty acids, and glucose levels in the pigeon, *Prostaglandins,* 8, 303, 1974

165.   Dray, F., Kouznetzova, B., Harris, B., and Brazeau, P., Role of prostaglandins on growth hormone secretion, *Adv Prostaglandin Thromboxane Res ,* 8, 1321, 1980.

166.   Rudofsky, G., The effect of intra-arterial and intravenous prostaglandin E₁ in a model of ischemia in healthy volunteers, in *Prostaglandin E₁ in Atherosclerosis,* Sinzinger, H and Rogatti, W., Eds., Springer-Verlag, New York, 1986, 49

167.   Creutzig, A., Caspany, L., and Alexander, K., Prospective open pilot study to investigate the efect of intermittent intra-arterial infusion treatment with prostaglandin E₁ in patients with intermittent claudication, in *Prostaglandin E₁ in Atherosclerosis,* Sinzinger, H. and Rogatti, W., Eds , Springer-Verlag, New York, 1986, 57.

168.   Gruss, J. D., Experiences with PGE₁ in patients with phlegmasia coerulea dolens and in ergotism, in *Prostaglandin E₁ in Atherosclerosis,* Sinzinger, H and Rogatti, W., Eds., Springer-Verlag, New York, 1986, 99.

169   Smith, J. B., Adam, I., Ingerman-Wojenshki, C. M., Siegl, A. M., and Silver, M. J., Prostaglandins as modulators of platelet function, in *Cardiovascular Pharmacology of Prostaglandins,* Herman, A G., Ed , Raven Press, New York, 1982, 115

170.   Sinzinger, H. and Rogatti, W., Eds., *Prostaglandin E₁ in Atherosclerosis,* Springer-Verlag, New York, 1986

171.   Sears, B., *BIOSYN Training Manual,* BIOSYN, Marblehead, MA, 1990.

172.   Brilla, L. R. and Landerholm, T. E., Effect of fish oil supplementation and exercise on serum lipids and aerobic fitness, *J Sports Med ,* 30(2), 173, 1990

173   Babayan, V. K., Medium-chain triglycerides — their composition, preparation, and application, *J Am Oil Chem Soc ,* 45, 23, 1967

174   Bach, A. S. and Babayan, V. K., Medium-chain triglycerides — an update, *Am J Clin Nutr ,* 36, 950, 1982.

175   Dupont, J., Lipids, in *Present Knowledge in Nutrition,* Brown, M. L., Ed , International Life Sciences Institute — Nutrition Foundation, Washington, D C , 1990, 56.

176   Seaton, T. B., Welle, S. L., Warenko, M. K., and Campbell, R. G., Thermic effect of medium-chain and long-chain triglycerides in man, *Am J Clin Nutr ,* 44, 630, 1986

177   Geliebter, A., Torbay, N., Bracco, E. F., Hashim, S. A., and van Itallie, T. B., Overfeeding with medium-chain triglyceride diet results in diminished deposition of fat, *Am J Clin Nutr ,* 37, 1, 1983

178   Baba, N., Bracco, E. F., and Hashim, S.A., Enhanced thermogenesis and diminished deposition of fat in response to overfeeding with diet containing medium chain triglyceride, *Am J Clin Nutr ,* 35, 678, 1982

179   Scalfi, L., Coltorti, A., and Contaldo, F., Postprandial thermogenesis in lean and obese subjects after meals supplemented with medium-chain and long-chain triglycerides, *Am J Clin Nutr ,* 53, 1130, 1991

180   Johnson, R. C., Young, S. K., Cotter, R., Lin, L., and Rowe, W. B., Medium-chain-triglyceride lipid emulsion: metabolism and tissue distribution, *Am J Clin Nutr ,* 52, 502, 1990

181   Hill, J. O., Peters, J. C., Yang, D., Sharp, T., Kaler, M., Abumrad, N. N., and Greene, H. L., Thermogenesis in human overfeeding with medium-chain triglycerides, *Metabolism,* 38, 641, 1989.

182. **Kaunitz, H., Slanetz, C. A., Johnson, R. E., Babayan, V. K., and Barsky, G.,** Relation of saturated, medium- and long-chain triglycerides to growth, appetite, thirst and weight maintenance requirements, *J Nutr*, 64, 513, 1958.

183 **Dias, V.,** Effects of feeding and energy balance in adult humans, *Metabolism*, 39, 887, 1990

184 **Blackburn, G. L., Kater, G., Mascioli, E. A., Kowalchuk, M., Babayan, V. K., and Bistrian, B. R.,** A reevaluation of coconut oil's effect on serum cholesterol and atherogenesis, *J Phil Med Assoc*, 65(1), 144, 1989.

185 **Csik, L. and Bencsik, J.,** Versuche uber die Wirkung von Vitamin B auf die Arbeitsleistung des Menschen Festzustellen, *Klin Wochenschr*, 6, 2275, 1927.

186 **Muller, C.,** Untersuchungen uber den Einfluss von Leberpraparaten auf dem Arbeitsstoffwechsel des Menschen, *Biochem Ztschr*, 216, 85, 1929

187 **Hano, U.,** Uber die pharmakodynamischen Eigenschaften des Vitamin B1, *Acad Polond*, *Cl Med*, 416, 203, 1937

188 **Minz, B. and Agid, R.,** Influence de la vitamin B1 sur l'activité de l'acetylcholine, *Compt Rend Acad Sci*, 205, 576, 1937

189 **Briem, H. J.,** Ermüdungsverzogerung durch vitamin B1, *Pflueger's Arch*, 242, 450, 1939.

190 **Gounelle, H.,** Action de la vitamin B1 dans l'exercise musculaire et la prevention de la fatigue, *Bull Soc Med Hop (Paris)*, 56, 255, 1940

191 **McCormick, W.,** Vitamin B_1 and physical endurance, *Med Rec*, 152, 439, 1940

192 **Morell, T.,** Ermüdungsbekämpfung durch körpereigene Wirkstoffe, *Dtsch Med Wochenschr*. 66, 398, 1940

193 **Williams, R. D., Mason, H. L., Wilder, R. M., and Smith, B. F.,** Observations on induced thiamine (vitamin B1) deficiency in man, *Arch Int Med*, 66, 786, 1940

194 **Droese, W.,** Über den Einfluss von B1-Traubenzuckerkombination auf die körperliche Leistungsfähigkeit und einen funktionellen Nachweiss von B1-Hypovitaminosen, *Munchen Med Wochenschr*, 88, 909, 1941

195 **Simonson, E., Enzer, N., Baer, A., und Draun, R.,** Influence of vitamin B (complex) surplus on capacity for muscular and mental work, *J Ind Hyg Toxicol*, 24, 83, 1942.

196 **Frankau, I. M.,** Acceleration of co-ordinated muscular effort by nicotinamide, *Br Med J*, 13, 601, 1943

197 **Kaiser, P.,** Über die Wirkung des vitamin B1 auf das isolierte Froschherz, *Pflueger's Arch*, 242, 504, 1939

198 **Keys, A.,** Physical performance in relation to diet, *Fed Proc*, 2, 164, 1943.

199 **Williams, M. H.,** The role of vitamins in physical activitiy, in *Nutritional Aspects of Human Physical and Athletic Performance*, 2nd ed., Charles C Thomas, Springfield, IL, 1985, 147

200 **Williams, M. H.,** Vitamin supplementation and athletic performance, *Int J Vitam Nutr Res*, Suppl 30, 163, 1989.

201 **Foltz, E. E., Ivy, A. C., and Barborka, C. J.,** Influence of components of the vitamin B complex on recovery from fatigue, *J Lab Clin Med*, 27, 1396, 1942.

202 **Karpovich, P. V. and Millman, N.,** Vitamin B1 and endurance, *N Engl J Med*, 226, 881, 1942

203 **Keys, A. and Henschel, A. F.,** Vitamin supplementation of U S Army rations in relation to fatigue and the ability to do muscular work, *J Nutr*, 23, 259, 1942.

204 **Archdeacon, J. W. and Murlin, J. R.,** The effect of thiamine depletion and restoration of muscular efficiency and endurance, *J Nutr*, 28, 241, 1944.

205 **Henschel, A., Taylor, H. L., Mickelsen, O., Brozek, J. M., and Keys, A.,** The effect of high vitamin C and B vitamin intakes on the ability of man to work in hot environments, *Fed Proc*, 3, 18, 1944

206. **Knippel, M., Mauri, L., Belluschi, R., Bana, G., Galli, C., Pusterla, G. L., Spreafico, M., and Troina, E.,** The action of thiamin on the production of lactic acid in cyclists, *Med Sport*, 39(1), 11, 1986

207 **Haralambie, G.,** Vitamin B2 status in athletes and the influence of riboflavin administration on neuromuscular irritability, *Nutr Metab*, 20, 1, 1976

208   Carlson, L., Havel, R., and Ekelund, L., Effect of nicotinic acid on the turnover rate and oxidation of the free fatty acids of plasma during exercise, *Metabolism*, 12, 837, 1963

209   Jenkins, D., Effects on nicotinic acid on carbohydrate and fat metabolism during exercise, *Lancet*, 1, 1307, 1965.

210   Norris, B., Schade, D. S., and Eaton, R. P., Effects of altered free fatty acid mobilization on the metabolic response to exercise, *J Clin Endocrinol Metab*, 46, 254, 1978.

211. Bergstrom, J., Hultman, E., Jorfeldt, L., Pernow, B., and Wahren, J., Effect of nicotinic acid on physical working capacity and on metabolism of muscle glycogen in man, *J Appl Physiol*, 26, 170, 1969

212   Pernow, B. and Saltin, B., Availability of substrates and capacity for prolonged heavy exercise in man, *J Appl Physiol*, 31, 416, 1971.

213. Lawrence, J., Smith, J., Bower, R., and Riehl, W., The effect of alpha-tocopherol (vitamin E) and pyridoxine HCl (vitamin B6) on the swimming endurance of trained swimmers, *J. Am Coll Health Assoc.*, 23, 219, 1974.

214   Marconi, C., Sassi, G., and Cerretalli, P., The effect of an alphaketoglutarate-pyridoxine complex on human maximal aerobic performance, *Eur J Appl Physiol*, 49, 307, 1982

215   Moretti, C., Fabbri, A., Gnessi, L., Bonifacio, V., Fraioli, F., and Isidori, A., Pyridoxine (B6) suppresses the rise in prolactin and increases the rise in growth hormone induced by exercise, *N Engl J Med*, 307(7), 444, 1982.

216   deVos, A. M., Leklem, J. E., and Campbell, D. E., Carbohydrate loading, vitamin B6 supplementation, and fuel metabolism during exercise in man, *Med Sci Sports Exer*, 14, 137, 1982.

217   Manore, M. M. and Leklem, J. E., Effect of carbohydrate and vitamin B6 on fuel substrates during exercise in women, *Med Sci Sports Exer*, 20, 233, 1988

218   Montoye, H., Spata, P., Pinckney, V., and Barron, L., Effects of vitamin B12 supplementation on physical fitness and growth of young boys, *J Appl Physiol*, 7, 589, 1955.

219   Montoye, H., Vitamin B12: a review, *Res Q Am Assoc Health Phys Ed*, 26, 308, 1955

220   Tin-May-Than, Ma-Win-May, Khin-Sann-Aung, and Mya-Tu, M., The effect of vitamin B12 on physical performance capacity, *Br J Nutr.*, 40, 269, 1978

221   Ellis, F. R. and Nasser, S., A pilot study of vitamin B12 in the treatment of tiredness, *Br J Nutr*, 30, 277, 1973.

222   Windholz, M., Ed., Cobamamide, in *The Merck Index*, 10th ed., Merck Co, Rahway, NJ, 1983, 348.

223   Roundtable, Popularized ergogenic aids, *NSCA J*, 11(1), 10, 1989

224   Wagner, J. C., Use of chromium and cobamamide by athletes, *Clin Pharm*, 8, 832, 1989

225   Stpopzyk, K., K., Kobalin — a new anabolic drug from the coenzyme group, *Przaglad Lekarski*, 25, 723, 1969.

226   Matter, M., Stittfall, R., Graves, J., Myburgh, K., Adams, B., Jacobs, P., and Noakes, T. D., The effect of iron and folate therapy on maximal exercise performance in female marathon runners with iron and folate deficiency, *Clin Sci*, 72, 415, 1987.

227   Nice, C., Reeves, A. G., Brinck-Johnsen, T., and Noll, W., The effects of pantothenic acid on human exercise capacity, *J Sports Med.*, 24, 26, 1984

228   Litoff, D., Scherzer, H., and Harrison, J., Effects of pantothenic acid supplementation on human exercise, *Med Sci. Sports Exer*, 17, 287, 1985.

229   Keys, A., Henschel, A., Taylor, H. L., Mickelsen, O., and Brozek, J., Experimental studies on man with a restricted intake of the B vitamins, *Am J Physiol*, 144, 5, 1945

230   Early, R. G. and Carlson, R. B., Water-soluble vitamin therapy in the delay of fatigue from physical activity in hot climatic conditions, *Int Z Angew Physiol.*, 27, 43, 1969

231. Bonke, D. and Nickel, B., Improvement of fine motoric movement control by elevated dosages of vitamin B_1, B_6, and B_{12} in target shooting, *Int J Vitam Nutr Res*, Suppl 30, 198, 1989.

232. van der Beek, E. J., van Dokkum, W., Schrijver, J., Wedel, M., Gaillard, A. W. K., Wesstra, A., van de Weerd, H., and Hermus, R. J. J., Thiamin, riboflavin, and vitamins B-6 and C: impact of combined restricted intake on functional performance in man, *Am J Clin Nutr*, 48, 1451, 1988

233 Buzina, R., Grgic, A., Jusic, M., Sapunar, J., Milanovic N., and Brubacher, G., Nutritional status and physical working capacity, *Hum Nour Clin Nutr* , 36C, 429, 1982
234 Fuijiwara, M., Allithiamine and its properties, *J Nutr Sci Vitaminol* , 22 (Suppl.), 57, 1976
235. Thomson, A. D., Frank, O., Baker, H., and Leevy, C. M., Thiamine propyldisulfide: adsorption and utilization, *Ann Int Med* , 74, 529, 1971
236 Baker, H. and Frank, O., Absorption, utilization and clinical effectiveness of allithiamines compared to water-soluble thiamines, *J Nutr Sci Vitaminol* , 22 (Suppl.), 63, 1976.
237 Lonsdale, D., Thiamine and its fat soluble derivatives as therapeutic agents, *Int Clin Nutr Rev* , 7(3), 114, 1987
238 Branca, D., Scutari, G., and Siliprandi, N., Pantethine and pantothenate effect on the CoA content of rat liver, *Int J Vitam Nutr Res* , 54, 211, 1984
239. Hyashi, H., Kobayashi, A., Terada, H., Nagao, B., Nishiyama, T., Kamikawa, T., and Yamakazi, N., Effects of pantethine on action potential of canine papillary muscle during hypoxic perfusion, *Jpn Heart J* , 26, 289, 1985
240 Minami, M., Yasuda, H., and Saito, H., Positive inotropic and negative chronotropic effect of pantethine on isolated cardiac muscle of guinea-pigs, *Experientia*, 39, 1028, 1983.
241 Shibano, T. and Abiko, Y., Effect of pantethine on myocardial pH reduced by partial occlusion of the coronary artery in dogs with special reference to the myocardial levels of adenosine triphosphate, creatine phosphate, and lactate, *Arch Int Pharmacodyn* , 255, 281, 1982.
242 Arsenio, L., Caronna, S., Lateana, M., Magnati, G., Strata, A., and Zammarchi, G., Hyperlipidemia, diabetes and atherosclerosis: efficacy of the treatment with pantethine, *Acta Biomed Ateneo Parmense*, 55, 25, 1984
243 Murai, A., Miyahara, T., Tanaka, T., Sako, Y., Mishimura, N., and Kameyama, M., The effects of pantethine on lipid and lipoprotein abnormalities in survivors of cerebral infarction, *Artery*, 12, 234, 1983
244. Miccoli, R., Marchett, P., Sampietro, T , Benzi, L., Tognarelli, M., and Navalesi, T., Effects of pantethine on lipids and apolipoproteins in hypercholesterolemic diabetic and nondiabetic patients, *Curr Ther Res* , 36, 545, 1984
245. Angelico, M., Pinto, G., Ciaccheri, C., Alvaro, D., De Santis, A., Marin, M., and Attili, A. F., Improvement in serum lipid profile in hyperlipoproteinaemic patients after treatment with pantethine: a cross-over, double-blind trial versus placebo, *Curr Ther Res* , 33, 1091, 1983
246. Wittwer, C. T., Gahl, W. A., Butler, J. D., Zatz, M., and Thoene, J. G., Metabolism of pantethine in cystinosis, *J Clin Invest* , 76, 1665, 1985
247 Williams, M. H., Vitamin, iron and calcium supplementation: effect on human physical performance, in *Nutrition and Athletic Performance*, Haskell, W , Scala, J , and Whittam, J , Eds , Bull Publishing, Palo Alto, CA, 1982, 106
248 Sieburg, H., *Dtsch Med Wochenschr Beil Arzt Sport*, 3, 11, 1937
249 Rugg-Gunn, M. A., *J R Nav Med Serv* , 3, 199, 1938.
250 Boje, O., Doping: a study of the means employed to raise the level of performance in sport, *Bull Health Org., League of Nations*, 8, 439, 1939
251 Jetzler, A. and Hamer, C., Vitamin C — Bedarf die einmaliger sportlicher Dauerleistung, *Wien Med Wochenschr* , 89, 332, 1939.
252 Weibel, H., Untersuchungen über vitamin C belastungen bei Sportsstudentinnen, *Dtsch Med Wochenschr* , 65, 60, 1939.
253. Basu, N. M. and Ray, G. K., The effect of vitamin C on the incidence of fatigue in human muscles, *Ind J Med Res* , 28, 419, 1940.
254 Cluver, E. H., Nutritional research in the Union of South Africa, *Bull Health Org , League of Nations*, 9, 327, 1940
255. Fox, F. W., Dangerfield, L. F., Gottlich, S. F., and Jokl, E., Vitamin C requirements of native mine labourers, *Br Med J* , 2, 143, 1940
256. Brunner, H., Vitamin C und Armeesport Erfahrungen mit Redoxon am schweizerischen Armee-Wettmarsch in Frauenfeld, *Dtsch Med Wochenschr* , 71, 715, 1941

257   Steinhaus, A. M., Exercise, *Annu Rev Physiol*, 3, 695, 1941
258   Anon., Vitamin C prevents heat cramps and heat prostration, *Science Suppl*, 95, 12, 1942
259   Hoitink, A. W., *Ned Tijdschr Ceneeskd*, 86, 1183, 1942.
260   Holmes, H. N., Vitamin C in the war, *Science*, 96, 384, 1942.
261   DuPain, R. and Loutfi, M., Vitamin C et courbatures, *Rev Med Suisse Romande*, 63, 640, 1943
262   Henschel, A., Taylor, H. L., Brozek, J., Mickelsen, O., and Keys, A., Vitamin C and ability to work in hot environments, *Am J Trop. Med Hyg*, 24, 259, 1944
263.   Johnson, R. E., Sargent, F., and Robinson, P. F., Effects of variation in dietary vitamin C on the physical well-being of manual workers, *J Nutr*, 29, 155, 1945.
264   Hoitink, A. W. J. H., Vitamin C and work Studies on the influence of work and of vitamin C intake on the human organism, *Verh Ned Inst Prevenr Geneeskd*, 4, 176, 1946.
265   Hoitink, A. W. J. H., Researches on the influence of vitamin C administration on the mechanical efficiency of the human organism, *Acta Brev Neerl Physiol Pharmacol Microbiol*, 14, 62, 1946.
266.   Bourne, G. H., Vitamins and muscular exercise, *Br. J Nutr*, 2, 261, 1948.
267   Malmosoki, L., Stadler, E., and Nemessuri, M., *Sportarztl Prax*, 3/4, 125, 1960
268   Namyslowski, L., Observations concerning the influence of vitamin C on the physical fitness of sportsmen, *Sportarztl Prax*, 3, 118, 1960.
269   Prokop, L., The effect of natural vitamin C on oxygen utilization and metabolic efficiency, *N Z Arztl Fortbild*, 49, 448, 1960
270   Rasch, P., Arnheim, D., and Klafs, C., Effects of vitamin C supplementation on cross-country runners, *Sportarztl Prax*, 5, 10, 1962.
271   Margaria, R., Aghemo, P., and Rovelli, E., The effect of some drugs on maximum capacity of athletic performance in man, *Int Z Angew Physiol*, 20, 281, 1964.
272   Van Huss, W., What made the Russians run?, *Nutr Today*, 1, 20, 1966
273   Baker, E. M., Vitamin C requirements in stress, *Am J Clin Nutr*, 20, 583, 1967
274   Kirchoff, H. W., Über dem Einfluss von Vitamin C auf Energieverbrauch, Kreislauf- und Ventilationsgrossen im Belastungsversuch, *Nutr. Dieta*, 11, 184, 1969
275   Bailey, D. A., Carron, A. V., Teece, R. G., and Wehner, H., Effect of vitamin C supplementation upon the physiological response to exercise in trained and untrained subjects, *Int J Vitam Res.*, 40, 435, 1970
276   Horak, J., Zenisek, A., and Benesova, H., Ascorbic acid blood level prior to laboratory work and after: its relation to spiroergometric parameters in top-performance athletes, *Cas Lek Cesk*, 116, 679, 1977.
277   Inbar, O. and Bar-Or, O., The effect of intermittent warm up on 7 to 9-year-old boys, *Eur J Appl Physiol*, 34, 81, 1975
278   Keith, R. and Driskell, J., Lung function and treadmill performance of smoking and nonsmoking males receiving ascorbic acid supplements, *Am J Clin Nutr*, 36, 840, 1982
279   Hoogerweif, A. and Hoitink, A., The influence of vitamin C administration on the mechanical efficiency of the human organism, *Int. Z Angew Physiol*, 20, 164, 1963
280   Spioch, F., Kobza, R., and Mazur, B., Influence of vitamin C upon certain functional changes and the coefficient of mechanical efficiency in humans during physical effort, *Acta Physiol Pol*, 17, 204, 1966.
281   Gey, G. O., Cooper, K. H., and Bottenberg, R. A., Effect of ascorbic acid on endurance performance and athletic injury, *JAMA*, 211, 105, 1970.
282   Bailey, D. A., Carron, A. V., Teece, R. G., and Wehner, H. J., Vitamin C supplementation related to physiological response to exercise in smoking and nonsmoking subjects, *Am J Clin Nutr*, 23, 905, 1970
283   Howald, H., Segesser, B., and Korner, W. F., Ascorbic acid and athletic performance, *Ann N Y Acad Sci*, 258, 458, 1975
284   Bender, A. and Nash, A., Vitamin C and physical performance, *Plant Foods for Men*, 1, 217, 1975
285   Inukai, M., The effect of vitamin C on anaerobic activities. Committee Report on Vitamin C, Japan Physical Education Association, No 5, 1977.

286. **Keren, G. and Epstein, Y.,** The effect of high dosage vitamin C intake on aerobic and anaerobic capacity, *J Sports Med* , 20, 145, 1980.

287 **Keith, R. E. and Merrill, E.,** The effects of vitamin C on maximum grip strength and muscular endurance, *J Sports Med* , 23, 253, 1983

288. **Bramich, K. and McNaughton, L.,** The effects of two levels of ascorbic acid on muscular endurance, muscular strength and on VO₂max, *Int Clin Nutr Rev* , 7, 5, 1987

289 **Suboticanec-Buzina, K., Buzina, R., Brubacher, G., Sapunar, J., and Christeller, S.,** Vitamin C status and physical working capacity in adolescents, *Int J Vitam Nutr Res* , 54, 55, 1984

290 **Som, S., Raha, C., and Chatterjee, I. B.,** Ascorbic acid: a scavenger of superoxide radical, *Acta Vitaminol Enzymol* , 5, 243, 1983

291 **Jaffe, G. M.,** Vitamin C, in *Handbook of Vitamins: Nutritional, Biochemical, and Clinical Aspects,* Machlin, L J , Ed., Marcel Dekker, New York, 1984, 199

292 **Olson, J.A.,** Vitamin A, in *Handbook of Vitamins: Nutritional, Biochemical, and Clinical Aspects,* Machlin, L J , Ed., Marcel Dekker, New York, 1984, 1.

293 **Anon.,** Russians research food requirements of athletes, *Swim Tech* , 8, 59, 1971

294 **Wald, G., Brouha, L., and Johnson, R.,** Experimental human vitamin A deficiency and ability to perform muscular exercise, *Am J Physiol* , 137, 551, 1942.

295 **Korner, W. F. and Vollm, J.,** New aspects of the tolerance of retinol in humans, *Int J Vitam Nutr Res* , 45, 363, 1975

296 **Fumich, R. and Essig, G.,** Hypervitaminosis. A case report in an adolescent soccer player, *Am J Sports Med* , 11, 37, 1983

297 **Krinsky, N. I. and Denke, S. M.,** The interaction of oxygen and oxyradicals with carotenoids, *J Natl. Canc Inst* , 69, 205, 1982.

298 **Richards, S. R., Chang, F. E., Bossetti, B., Malarkey, W. B., and Kim, M. H.,** Serum carotene levels in female long-distance runners, *Fertil Steril* , 43, 79, 1985.

299 **Olson, J.A.,** Vitamin A, in *Present Knowledge in Nutrition,* Brown, M. L., Ed., International Life Sciences Institute — Nutrition Foundation, Washington, D C., 1990, 96.

300 **Mathews-Roth, M. M.,** Plasma concentrations of carotenoids after large doses of β-carotene, *Am J Clin Nutr* , 52, 500, 1990.

301 **Norman, A. W. and Miller, B. E.,** Vitamin D, in *Handbook of Vitamins: Nutritional, Biochemical, and Clinical Aspects,* Machlin, L. J., Ed , Marcel Dekker, New York, 1984, 45

302 **Seidl, E. and Hettinger, T.,** Der Einfluss von Vitamin D3 auf Kraft und Leistungsfähgkeit des gesunden Erwachsenen, *Int Z Angew Physiol* , 16, 365, 1957

303 **Berven, H.,** The physical working capacity of healthy children. Seasonal variation and effect of ultraviolet radiation and vitamin D supply, *Acta Pediatr* , 148 (Suppl), 1, 1963.

304 **Machlin, L. J., Ed.,** *Vitamin E A Comprehensive Treatise,* Marcel Dekker, New York, 1984

305 **Diplock, A. T.,** Vitamin E, selenium and free radicals, *Med Biol* , 62, 78, 1984

306 **Shephard, R. J.,** Vitamin E and athletic performance, *J Sports Med* , 23, 461, 1983.

307 **Cureton, T. K., Ed.,** *The Physiological Effects of Wheat Germ Oil on Humans in Exercise.* Charles C Thomas, Springfield, IL, 1972.

308 **Aoki, J., Shimiu, T., and Maeshima, T.,** Effect of vitamin E and C compound as ergogenic aids to physiological response of male long distance runners in physical training programs, *Bull Sch Phys Ed Juntendo Univ* , 12, 14, 1969.

309 **Cureton, T. K.,** Effect of wheat germ oil and vitamin E on normal human subjects in physical training programs, *Am J Physiol* , 179, 628, 1954

310 **Clausen, D.,** The Combined Effect of Aerobic Exercise and Vitamin E upon Cardiorespiratory Endurance and Measured Blood Variables, Master's thesis, University of Wyoming, Cheyenne, 1971.

311 **Cureton, T. K.,** Wheat germ oil, the "wonder" fuel, *Scholastic Coach,* 24, 36, 1955

312 **Nagawa, T., Kita, H., Aoki, J., Maeshima, T., and Shiozawa, K.,** The effect of vitamin E on endurance, *Asian Med J* , 11, 619, 1968

313   Kobayashi, Y., Effect of Vitamin E on Aerobic Work Performance in Man During Acute Exposure to Hypoxic Hypoxia, Ph D dissertation, University of New Mexico, Albuquerque, 1974.

314   Prokop, L., Die Wirkung von naturlichem Vitamin E auf Sauerstoffverbrauch und Sauerstoffschuld, *Sportarztl. Prax*, 1, 19, 1960

315   Ogawa, S., Effect of vitamin E and vitamin C compound on aerobic physical performance in a cold environment. Report of Sports Sci Res., Jpn. Amat. Sports Assoc., 1970, 1

316   Sakaeva, E. and Efremov, V., Experience with additional allowance of vitamin E to sportsmen-race cyclists and skiers, *Vestn Akad Med Nauk. S S S R*, 27, 78, 1972.

317   Efremov, V. and Sakaeva, E., Importance of vitamin E in intense physical exertions of sportsmen, *Vopr Pitan*, 32, 22, 1973

318   Percival, L., Vitamin E in athletic efficiency (preliminary report), *The Summary*, 3, 55, 1951

319. Shute, E. V., Vitamin E for athletes, *The Summary*, 23, 3, 1971

320   Simon-Schnazz, I. and Pabst, H., Influence of vitamin E on physical performance, *Int J Vitam Nutr Res*, 58, 49, 1988.

321   Dillard, C. J., Litov, R. E., Savin, W. M., Dumelin, E. E., and Tappel, A. L., Effects of exercise, vitamin E and ozone on pulmonary function and lipid peroxidation, *J Appl Physiol*, 45, 927, 1978

322   Goldfarb, A. H., Todd, M. K., Boyer, B. T., Alessio, H. M., and Cutler, R. G., Effect of vitamin E on lipid peroxidation at 80% VO_2max, *Med Sci Sports Exer*, 21(2), S16, 1989

323   Sumida, S., Tanaka, K., Kitao, H., and Nakadamo, F., Exercise-induced lipid peroxidation and leakage of enzymes before and after vitamin E supplementation, *Int J Biochem*, 21, 835, 1989

324   Belakovskii, M. S. and Bogdanov, N. G., Vitamins during adaption to high altitudes, *Kosm Biol Aviakosm Med*, 18, 4, 1984.

325   Hove, E. L., Hickman, K. C. D., and Harris, P. L., The effect of tocopherol and of fat on the resistance of rats to anoxic anoxia, *Arch Biol Chem*, 8, 395, 1945

326   Kamimura, M., Takahashi, S., and Henmi, I., On the influence of vitamin E on the low oxygen tolerance of mice, *Sapporo Med J*, 21, 71, 1962

327   Telford, I. R., Wiswell, O. B., and Smith, E. L., Tocopherol prophylaxis in multiple exposure to hypoxia, *Proc Soc Exp Biol Med*, 87, 162, 1954.

328   Lawrence, J., Bower, R., Riehl, W., and Smith, J., Effects of alpha-tocopherol acetate on the swimming endurance of trained swimmers, *Am J Clin Nutr*, 28, 205, 1974.

329. Sharman, I. M., Down, M. G., and Sen, R. N., The effects of vitamin E and training on physiological function and athletic performance in adolescent swimmers, *Br J Nutr*, 26, 265, 1971.

330   Sharman, I. M., Down, M. G., and Morgan, N. G., The effects of vitamin E on physiological function and athletic performance of trained swimmers, *J Sports Med*, 16, 215, 1976.

331   Shephard, R. J., Campbell, R., Pimm, P., Stuart, D., and Wright, G., Vitamin E, exercise and the recovery from physical activity, *Eur J Appl Physiol*, 33, 119, 1974

332   Shephard, R. J., Stuart, R., Campbell, R., Wright, G., and Pimm, P., Do athletes need vitamin E?, *Phys Sportsmed*, 2, 57, 1974

333   Talbot, D. and Jamieson, J., An examination of the effect of vitamin E on the performance of highly trained swimmers, *Can J Appl Sci*, 2, 67, 1977.

334   Watt, T., Romet, T. T., McFarlane, L., McGuey, D., Allen, C., and Goode, R. C., Vitamin E and oxygen consumption, *Lancet*, 2, 354, 1974

335   Mayer, J. and Bullen, B., Nutrition and athletic performance, *Postgrad Med*, 26, 848, 1959

336   Helgheim, I., Hetland, O., Nilsson, S., Ingjer, F., and Stromme, S. B., The effects of vitamin E on serum enzyme levels following heavy exercise *Eur J Appl Physiol*, 40, 283, 1979

337 Bunnell, R. H., De Ritter, E., and Rubin, S. H., Effect of feeding polyunsaturated fatty acids with a low vitamin E diet on blood levels of tocopherol in men performing hard physical labor, *Am J Clin Nutr*, 28, 706, 1975.

338 Hackney, J. D., Linn, W. S., Buckley, R. D., Jones, M. P., Wightman, L. H., Karuza, S. K., Blessey, R. L., and Hislop, H. J., Vitamin E supplementation and respiratory effects of ozone in humans. *J Toxicol Environ Health*, 7, 383, 1981

339 Shephard, R. J., Athletic performance and urban air pollution, *Can Med Assoc J*, 131, 105, 1984

340 Novelli, G. P., Bracciotti, G., and Falsini, S., Spin-trappers and vitamin E prolong endurance to muscle fatigue in mice, *Free Rad Biol Med.*, 8, 9, 1990.

341 Baker, H. D., Frank, B., DeAngelis, B., and Fiengold, S., Plasma tocopherol in man at various times after ingesting free or acetylated tocopherol, *Nutr Rep Int*, 21, 531, 1980

342 Horwitt, M. K., Elliot, W. H., Kanjananggulapan, P., and Fitch, C. D., Serum concentrations of alpha-tocopherol after ingestion of various vitamin E preparations, *Am J Clin Nutr*, 40, 240, 1984

343 Ogihara, T., Nishida, Y., Miki, M., and Mino, M., Comparative changes in plasma and RBC alpha-tocopherol after administration of dl-alpha-tocopheryl acetate and d-alpha-tocopherol, *J Nutr Sci Vitaminol*, 31, 169, 1985.

344 Losowsky, M. S., Kelleher, J., Walker, B. E., Davies, T., and Smith, C. L., Intake and absorption of tocopherol, *Ann NY Acad Sci*, 203, 212, 1972.

345 Schmandke, H. and Schmidt, G., Absorption of alpha-tocopherol from oily and aqueous solution, *Int J Vitam Nutr Res*, 35, 138, 1965.

346 Gerster, H., Function of vitamin E in physical exercise: a review, *Z Ernahrungswiss*, 30(2), 89, 1991.

347 Gee, D. L. and Tappel, A. L., The effect of exhaustive exercise on expired pentane as a measure of in vivo lipid peroxidation in the rat, *Life Sci.*, 28, 2425, 1981.

348 Suzuki, M., Katamine, S., and Tatsumi, S., Exercise-induced enhancement of lipid peroxide metabolism in tissues and their transference into the brain in rat, *J Nutr Sci Vitaminol*, 29, 141, 1983.

349 Packer, L., Vitamin E, physical exercise and tissue damage in animals, *Med Biol.*, 62, 105, 1984

350 Packer, L., Mitochondria, oxygen radicals and animal exercise, in *Membr Muscle Proc Int Symp*, Berman, M. C., Gevers, W., and Opie, L. H., Eds, IRL Press, Oxford, 1985, 135

351 Suttie, J. W., Vitamin K, in *Handbook of Vitamins Nutritional, Biochemical and Clinical Aspects*, Machlin, L J, Ed., Marcel Dekker, New York, 1984, 147

352 Sahlin, K., Alvestrand, A., Brandt, R., and Hultman, E., Intracellular pH and bicarbonate concentration in human muscle during recovery from exercise, *J Appl Physiol*, 45, 474, 1978

353 Sahlin, K., Harris, R. C., and Hultman, E., Lactate content and pH in muscle samples obtained after dynamic exercise, *Pfluegers Arch*, 367, 143, 1976

354 Hultman, E. and Sahlin, K., Acid-base balance during exercise, *Exer Sport Sci Rev*, 8, 41, 1980

355 Williams, M. H., Ergogenic Foods (Aklaline Salts), in *Nutritional Aspects of Human Physical and Athletic Performance*, 2nd ed, Charles C Thomas, Springfield, IL, 1985, 297

356 Danforth, W. H., Activation of glycolytic pathway in muscle, in *Control of Energy Metabolism*, Chance, B and Estabrook, R. W., Eds, Academic Press, New York, 1965

357 Ui, M., A role of phosphofructokinase in pH-dependent regulation of glycolysis, *Biochem Biophys Acta*, 124, 310, 1966

358 Dennig, H., Peters, K., and Schneikert, O., Die Beeinflussung köperlieher Arbeit durch Azidose und Alkalose, *Arch Exp Path Pharmakol*, 165, 161, 1932.

359 Hewitt, J. and Callaway, E., Alkali reserve of the blood in relation to swimming performance, *Res Q Am Assoc Health Phys Ed*, 7, 83, 1936

360   **Jones, N. L., Sutton, J. R., Lin, J., Ward, G., Richardson, W., and Toews, C. J.,** Effects of acidosis on exercise performance and muscle glycolysis in man, *Clin Res* , 23, 636A, 1976

361   **Sutton, J. R., Jones, N. L., and Toews, C. J.,** Growth hormone secretion in acid-base alterations at rest and during exercise, *Clin Sci Mol Med* , 50, 241, 1976.

362   **Jones, N. L., Sutton, J. R., Taylor, R., and Toews, C. J.,** Effect of pH on cardiorespiratory and metabolic responses to exercise, *J Appl Physiol* , 43, 959, 1977.

363   **Kostka, C. E. and Cafarelli, E.,** Effect of pH on sensation during cycling exercise, *Med Sci Sports Exer* , 13, 85, 1981.

364   **Ehrsam, R. E., Heigenhauser, G. J. F., and Jones, N. L.,** The effect of respiratory acidosis on metabolism in exercise, *Med Sci. Sports Exer* , 12, 112, 1980.

365   **Sutton, J. R., Jones, N. L., and Toews, C. J.,** Effect of pH on muscle glycolysis during exercise, *Clin Sci* , 61, 331, 1981.

366   **Kowalchuk, J. M., Heigenhauser, G. J. F., and Jones, N. L.,** The effect of acid-base disturbances on ventilatory and metabolic responses to progressive exercise, *Med Sci Sports Exer* , 15, 111, 1983.

367   **McCartney, N., Heigenhauser, G. J. F., and Jones, N. L.,** Effects of pH on maximal power output and fatigue during short-term dynamic exercise, *J Appl Physiol.*, 55, 225, 1983.

368   **Dennig, H., Talbott, J. H., Edwards, H. T., and Dill, D. B.,** Effect of acidosis and alkalosis upon capacity for work, *J Clin Invest* , 9, 601, 1931.

369   **Dill, D. B., Edwards, H. T., and Talbott, J. H.,** Alkalosis and the capacity for work, *J Biol Chem* , 97, lviii, 1932

370   **Margaria, R., Edwards, H. T., and Dill, D. B.,** The possible mechanisms of contracting and paying the oxygen debt and the role of lactic acid in muscular contraction, *Am J Physiol* , 106, 689, 1933.

371   **Dennig, H.,** Über Steigerung der körperlichen Leistungsfähigkeit durch Eingriffe in den Säurebasenhaushalt, *Dtsch Med Wochenschr* , 63, 733, 1937.

372   **Dennig, H., Becker-Fregseng, H., Rendenbach, R., and Schostak, G.,** Leistungssteigerung in künstlicher Alkalose bei wiederholter Arbeit, *Naunyn-Schmied Arch* , 195, 261, 1940

373   **Dorow, H., Galuba, B., Hellwig, H., and Becker-Freyseng, H.,** Der Einfluss künstlicher Alkalose auf die sportliche Leistung von Laufern und Schwimmern, *Naunyn-Schmied Arch* , 195, 264, 1940.

374   **Parade, G. W. and Otto, H.,** Alkali-Reserve und Leistung, *Z Klin Med* , 137, 7, 1939

375   **Karpovich, P.,** Ergogenic aids in work and sports, *Res Q Suppl* , 12, 432, 1941.

376   **Johnson, W. R. and Black, D. H.,** Comparison of effects of certain blood alkalinizers and glucose upon competitive endurance performance, *J Appl. Physiol* , 5, 577, 1953.

377   **Linderman, J. and Fahey, T. D.,** Sodium bicarbonate ingestion and exercise performance An update, *Sports Med* , 11(2), 71, 1991.

378   **Margaria, R., Aghemo, P., and Sassi, G.,** Effect of alkalosis on performance and lactate formation in supramaximal exercise, *Int Z Angew. Physiol* , 29, 215, 1971.

379. **Simmons, R. and Hardt, A.,** The effect of alkali ingestion on the performance of trained swimmers, *J Sports Med.*, 13, 159, 1973

380   **Inbar, O., Rotstein, A., Jacobs, I., Kaiser, P., Dlin, R., and Dotan, R.,** Effect of induced alkalosis on short maximal exercise performance, *Med. Sci Sports Exer* , 13, 128, 1981.

381   **Grassi, M., Messuna, B., Fraiolo, A., Schietroma, M., Giacomo, M. L. D., and Grossi, F.,** Effects of bicarbonate-alkaline earth water (Sangemini) on some parameters of blood chemistry in wrestlers after exertion, *J Sports Med* , 23, 102, 1983.

382. **Wilkes, D., Gledhill, N., Smyth, R., and Tomlinson, J.,** The effect of acute induced metabolic alkalosis on anaerobic performance, *Med Sci. Sports Exer* , 13, 85, 1981

383. **Robertson, R., Falkel, J., Drash, A., Spungen, S., Metz, K., Swank, A., and LeBoeuf, J.,** Effect of induced alkalosis on differentiated perceptions of exertion during arm and leg movement, *Med Sci Sports Exer* , 14, 158, 1982

384 Costill, D. L., Verstappen, F., Kuipers, H., Jansson, E., and Funk, W., Acid-base balance during repeated bouts of exercise: influence of HCO_3^-, *Med Sci Sports Exer*, 15, 115, 1983

385 Rupp, J. C., Bartels, R. L., Zuelzer, W., Fox, E. L., and Clark, R. N., Effect of sodium bicarbonate ingestion on blood and muscle pH and exercise performance, *Med. Sci Sports Exer*, 15, 115, 1983.

386 Wilkes, D., Gledhill, N., and Smyth, R., Effect of acute induced metabolic alkalosis on 800-m racing time, *Med Sci Sports Exer*, 15, 277, 1983

387 Costill, D. L., Verstappen, F., Kuipers, H., Janssen, E., and Fink, W., Acid-base balance during repeated bouts of exercise: influence of HCO_3, *Int J Sports Med*, 5, 228, 1984

388 Horewill, C. A., Gao, J., and Costill, D. L., Oral $NaHCO_3$ improves performance in interval swimming, *Med Sci Sports Exer*, 20, S3, 1988

389 Pfefferle, K. P. and Wilkinson, J. G., Induced alkalosis and supramaximal cycling in trained and untrained men, *Med Sci Sports Exer*, 20, 525, 1988

390 Bouissou, P., Defer, G., Guezennec, C. Y., Estrade, P. Y., and Serrurier, B., Metabolic and blood catecholamine responses to exercise in alkalosis, *Med Sci Sports Exer*, 20, 228, 1988

391 Messina, B., Cairella, M., Trasatti, M., and Vecchi, L., Azione della terapia con un'acqua bicarbonato-alcalino-terrosa (Sangemini) su alcuni aspetti della sindrome da affaticamento negli sportivi, *Clin Term*, 17, 227, 1964.

392 Messina, B., Cairella, M., Simonotti, P. L., and Vecchi, L., Comportamento di alcune costanti ematochimiche in corso di prova da sforzo negli sportivi, *Clin Term*, 17, 399, 1964.

393 Messina, B., Cairella, M., Nasta, G., Simonotti, P. L., and Vecchi, L., Osservazioni sul trattamento con acqua bicarbonato-alcalino-terrosa (Sangemini) in atleti in allenamento, *Med Sport*, 20, 690, 1966

394 Messina, B., Gruaol, M., Fraioli, A., Pellegrino, M. R., Di Giacomo, M. L., and Grossi, F., Variazioni enzimatiche sieriche in nuotatori dopo sforzo (influenza di un trattamento con acqua bicarbonato-alcalino-terrosa), *Med Sport*, 35, 121, 1982

395 Miscia, G., Modificazioni del dolore muscolare da sforzo indotte dalla somministrazione di un'acqua minerale bicarbonato-calcica, *Med Sport*, 37, 4, 1984.

396. Inbar, O., Rotstein, A., Jacobs, I., Kaiser, P., and Dlin R., The effects of alkaline treatment on short-term maximal exercise, *J Sport Sci.*, 1, 95, 1983.

397 McKenzie, D. C., Coutts, K. D., Stirling, D. R., Hoeben, H. H., and Kazara, G., Maximal work production following two levels of induced metabolic alkalosis, *J Sports Sci*, 4, 35, 1986

398 Parry-Billings, M. and MacLaren, D. P. M., The effect of sodium bicarbonate and sodium citrate ingestion on anaerobic power during intermittent exercise, *Eur J Appl Physiol*, 55, 524, 1986

399 Grassi, M., Fraioli, A., Messina, B., Mammucari, S., and Mennuni, G., Mineral waters in treatment of metabolic changes from fatigue in sportsmen, *J Sports Med*, 30(4), 441, 1990.

400 Karpovich, P. and Sinning, W., Eds., *Physiology of Muscular Activity*, W B. Saunders, Philadelphia, 1971, 264.

401 Poulus, A. J., Docter, H. J., and Westra, H. G., Acid-base balance and subjective feelings of fatigue during physical exercise, *Eur J Appl Physiol*, 33, 207, 1974

402 Kinderman, W., Keul, J., and Huber, G., Physical exercise after induced alkalosis (bicarbonate or Tris buffer), *Eur J Appl Physiol*, 37, 197, 1977

403 Hunter, C., Van Huss, W., Boosharga, K., Smoak, B., Ho, K., and Heusner, W., The effects of sodium bicarbonate and diet upon acid-base balance in exhaustive work of short duration, *Med Sci Sports Exer*, 12, 127, 1980

404 Balberman, S. E. and Roby, F. B., The effects of induced alkalosis and acidosis on the work capacity of the quadriceps and hamstrings muscle groups, *Int J Sports Med*, 4, 143, 1983

405. Katz, A., Costill, D. L., King, D. S., Hargreaves, M., and Fink, W. J., Effect of oral alkalizer on maximal exercise tolerance, *Med Sci. Sports Exer*, 15, 126, 1983.

406. Katz, A., Costill, D. L., King, D. S., Hargreaves, M., and Fink, W. J., Maximal exercise tolerance after induced alkalosis, *Int J Sports Med*, 5, 107, 1984

407. Wijnen, S., Verstappen, F., and Kuipers, H., The influence of intravenous $NaHCO_3$-administration on interval exercise: acid-base balance and endurance, *Int J Sports Med*, 5(Suppl.), 130, 1984

408. Robins, K. and Verity, L. S., Effect of induced alkalosis on rowing ergometer performance (REP) during repeated 1-mile workouts, *Med Sci Sports Exer.*, 19, S68, 1987

409 Klein, L., The effect of bicarbonate ingestion on upper body power in trained athletes, *Med Sci Sports Exer*, 19, S67, 1987

410. Hooker, S., Morgan, C., and Wells, C., Effect of sodium bicarbonate ingestion on time to exhaustion and blood lactate of 10K runners, *Med Sci. Sports Exer*, 19, S67, 1987

411 Horswill, C. A., Costill, D. L., Fink, W. J., Flynn, M. G., Kirwan, J. P., Mitchell, J. B., and Houmard, J. A., Influence of sodium bicarbonate on sprint performance: relationship to dosage, *Med Sci Sports Exer*, 20, 566, 1988

412 George, K. P. and MacLaren, D. P. M., The effect of induced alkalosis and acidosis on endurance running at an intensity corresponding to 4mM blood lactate, *Ergonomics*, 31(11), 1639, 1988

413. Davies, K. J. A., Quintanilha, A. T., Brooks, G. A., and Packer, L., Free radicals and tissue damage produced by exercise, *Biochem Biophys Res Commun.*, 107, 1198, 1982

414. Brady, P. S., Ku, P. K., and Ullrey, D. E., Lack of effect of selenium supplementation on the response of equine erythrocyte glutathione system and plasma enzymes to exercise, *Biochem Biophys Res Commun*, 107, 1198, 1982

415. Packer, L., Oxygen radicals and antioxidants in endurance exercise, in *Biochemical Aspects of Physical Exercise*, Benzi, G., Packer, L, and Siliprandi, N., Eds., Elsevier, Amsterdam, 1985, 73.

416. Kagan, V. E., Spirichev, V. B., and Erin, A. N., Vitamin E in physical exercise and sport, in *Nutrition in Exercise and Sport*, Hickson, J. F. and Wolinsky, I., Eds., CRC Press, Boca Raton, FL, 1989, 255

417. Sjödin, B., Westing, Y. H., and Apple, F. S., Biochemical mechanisms for oxygen free radical formation during exercise, *Sports Med*, 10(4), 236, 1990

418. Balke, P. O., Snider, M. T., and Bull, A. P., Evidence for lipid peroxidation during moderate exercise in man, *Med Sci Sports Exer*, 16, 181, 1984.

419. Blokha, V. V., Kagen, V. Y., Sitovskii, M. V., Danilov, V. S., Kol's, O. R., and Kozlov, Y. P., Peroxidation of lipids and conduction of excitation in frog muscles, *Biofizida*, 17, 549, 1972

420. Brady, P. S., Brady, L. J., and Ullrey, D. E., Selenium, vitamin E and the response to swimming stress in the rat, *J Nutr*, 109, 1103, 1979.

421. Jenkins, R. R., Martin, D., and Goldberg, E., Lipid peroxidation in skeletal muscle during atrophy and acute exercise, *Med Sci Sports Exer*, 16, 93, 1983

422. Salminen, A. and Vihko, V., Lipid peroxidation and exercise myopathy, *Exp Mol Pathol*, 38, 380, 1983

423. Wilhelm, J. and Sonka, J., Effects of sublethal gamma irradiation and exercise on succinate oxidase and metabolites of lipid peroxides. 11 Rat skeletal muscle, *Aggressologie*, 21, 87, 1980

424. Ullrey, D. E., Shelle, J. E., and Brady, P. S., Rapid response of the equine erythrocyte glutathione peroxidase system to exercise, *Fed Proc*, 36, 1095, 1977.

425. Dohm, G. L., Kasperek, G. J., Tapscott, E. B., and Beecher, G. R., Effect of exercise on synthesis and degradation of muscle protein, *Biochem J*, 188, 255, 1980

426. Hecht, H. J., Schumann, H. J., and Kunde, D., Histologische und enzymhistochemische Befunde am Skelettmuskel der utrainierten Ratte nach intensiver physischer Belastung, *Med Sport (Berlin)*, 15, 270, 1975

427. Salminen, A. and Vihko, V., Acid proteolytic capacity in mouse cardiac and skeletal muscle after prolonged submaximal exercise, *Pfluegers Arch*, 389, 17, 1980.

428   Vihko, V., Rantamaki, J., and Salminen, A., Exhaustive physical exercise and acid hydrolase activity in mouse skeletal muscle A histochemical study, *Histochemistry*, 57, 237, 1978

429   Vihko, V., Salminen, A., and Rantamaki, J., Acid hydrolase activity in red and white skeletal muscle of mice during a two-week period following exhaustive exercise, *Pfluegers Arch*, 378, 99, 1978

430   Jenkins, R. R., The role of superoxide dismutase and catalase in muscle fatigue, in *Biochemistry of Exercise Vol 13*, Knuttgen, H. G., Vogel, I. A., and Poortmans, J., Eds., Human Kinetics Publishers, Champaign, IL, 1983, 467.

431   Jenkins, R. R., Friedland, R., and Howald, H., The relationship of oxygen uptake to superoxide dismutase and catalase activity in human skeletal muscle, *Int J Sports Med*, 5, 11, 1984.

432   Higuchi, M., Cartier, L. J., and Holloszy, J. O., The effects of endurance training on free radical scavenging enzymes in rats, *Med Sci Sports Exer*, 15, 93, 1983

433   Salminen, A. and Vihko, V., Endurance training reduces the susceptibility of mouse skeletal muscle to lipid peroxidation, in vitro, *Acta Physiol Scand*, 117, 109, 1983.

434   Vihko, V., Salminen, A., and Rantamaki, J., Exhaustive exercise, endurance training, and acid hydrolase activity in skeletal muscle, *J Appl Physiol*, 47, 43, 1979

435   Corbucci, G. G., Montanari, G., Cooper, M. B., Jones, D. A., and Edwards, R. H. T., The effect of exertion on mitochondrial oxidative capacity and on some antioxidant mechanisms in muscle from marathon runners, *Int J Sports Med*, Suppl 5, 135, 1984.

436   Cannon, J. G. and Kluger, M. J., Endogenous pyrogen activity in human plasma after exercise, *Science*, 220, 617, 1983

437   Schaefer, R. M., Kokot, K., Heidland, A., and Plass, R., Jogger's leukocytes, *N Engl J Med*, 316, 223, 1987.

438   Beaman, L. and Beaman, B. L., The role of oxygen and its derivatives in microbial pathogenesis and host defense, *Annu Rev Microbiol*, 38, 27, 1984

439   Segal, A. W., How do phagocytic cells kill bacteria? *Med Biol*, 62, 81, 1984

440   Sepe, S. M. and Clark, R. A., Oxidant membrane injury by the neutrophil myeloperoxidase system. 1. Characterization of a liposome model and injury by myeloperoxidase, hydrogen peroxide, and halides, *J Immunol* 134, 1888, 1985.

441   Sevanian, A. and Hochstein, P., Mechanisms and consequences of lipid peroxidation in biological systems, *Annu Rev Nutr*, 5, 365, 1985

442. Meerson, F. Z., Krasikov, S. I., Boev, V. M., and Kagan, V. E., Effect of an antioxidant on the untrained body Resistance to maximal exercise, *Bull Exp Biol Med*, 94, 17, 1982

443   Viguie, C. A., Packer, L., and Brooks, G. A., Antioxidant supplementation affects indices of muscle trauma and oxidant stress in human blood during exercise, *Med Sci Sports Exer*, 21(2), S16, 1989

443a Singh, V. N., A current perspective on nutrition and exercise, *J Nutr*, 122, 760, 1992

443b Witt, E. H., Reznick, A. Z., Viguie, C. A., Starke-Reed, P., and Packer, L., Exercise, oxidative damage and effects of antioxidant manipulation, *J Nutr*, 122, 766, 1992

444   Ismail, A. H., Petro, T. M., and Watson, R. R., Dietary supplementation with vitamin E and C in fit and nonfit adults: biochemical and immunological changes, *Fed Proc*, 42, 335, 1983.

445   Bucci, L. R., Klenda, B. A., Stiles, J. C., and Sparks, W. S., Truth in labeling for antioxidant enzyme products Survey of label claims and product potencies, in *Proceedings, Second Symposium on Nutrition and Chiropractic*, Faruqui, S R and Ansari, M S, Eds., Palmer College of Chiropractic, Davenport, IA, 1989, 56

446   Ambrus, J. L., Lassman, B. A., and DeMarchi, J. J., Absorption of exogenous and endogenous proteolytic enzymes, *Clin Pharmacol Ther*, 8, 362, 1967

447   Avakian, S., Further studies on the absorption of chymotrypsin *Clin Pharmacol Ther*, 5, 712, 1964.

448   Izaka, K., Yamada, M., Lawano, T., and Suyama, T., Gastrointestinal absorption and anti-inflammatory effect of bromelain, *Jpn J Pharmacol*, 22, 519, 1972

449 Kabacoff, B. L., Wohlman, A., Umhey, M., and Avakian, S., Absorption of chymotrypsin from the intestinal tract, *Nature*, 199, 815, 1963.

450 Miller, J. M. and Opher, A. W., The increased proteolytic activity of human blood serum after the oral administration of bromelain, *Exp Med Surg*, 22, 277, 1964

451 Miller, J. M., The absorption of proteolytic enzymes from the gastrointestinal tract, *Clin Med*, 75, 35, 1968

452 Seifert, J., Ganser, R., and Brendel, W., Die Resorption eines proteolytischen Enzyms pflanzlichen Ursprunges aus dem Magen-Darmtrakt in das Blut und in die Lymphe von erwachsenen Ratten, *Z für Gastroenterol*, 17, 1, 1979.

453 Smyth, R. D., Brennan, R., and Martin, G. J., Studies establishing the absorption of the bromelains (proteolytic enzymes) from the gastrointestinal tract, *Exp Med Surg*, 22, 46, 1964

454. Giri, S. N. and Misra, H. P., Fate of superoxide dismutase in mice following oral route of administration *Med Biol*, 62, 285, 1984

455. Zidenburg-Cherr, S., Keen, C. L., Lonnerdal, B., and Hurley, L. S., Dietary superoxide dismutase does not affect tissue levels, *Am J Clin Nutr*, 37, 5, 1983

456. Walker, W. A., Cornell, R., Davenport, L. M., and Isselbacher, K. J., Macromolecular absorption: mechanism of horseradish peroxidase uptake and transport in adult and neonatal rat intestine, *J Cell Biol*, 54, 195, 1972.

457. Warshaw, A. L., Walker, W. A., Cornell, R., and Isselbacher, K. J., Small intestine permeability to macromolecules: transmission of horseradish peroxidase into mesenteric lymph and portal blood, *Lab Invest*, 25, 675, 1971

458 Baintner, K., Ed., *Intestinal Absorption of Macromolecules and Immune Transmission from Mother to Young*, CRC Press, Boca Raton, FL, 1986

459 Siakotos, A. N. and Armstrong, D., Age pigment, a biochemical indicator of intracellular aging, in *Neurobiology of Aging*, Ordy, J M and Brizze, K. R., Eds., Plenum Press, New York, 1975, 369

460 McGilvery, R. W., Ed., *Biochemistry A Functional Approach*, 2nd ed, W B. Saunders, Philadelphia, 1979, 566.

461 Nieper, H. A. and Blumberger, K., Electrolyte transport therapy of cardiovascular diseases, in *Electrolytes and Cardiovascular Diseases, Vol 2*, Bajusz, E, Ed, S. Karger, Basel, 1966, 141

462. Laborit, H., Maynier, R., Guiot, G., Barow, C., and Niaussat, P., Influence of various pharmacological agents on the swimming test of white rats, *Compt Rend Soc Biol*, 152, 486, 1958.

463 Laborit, H., Weber, B., Jouany, J., Niassat, R., and Barow, C., Metabolism of ammonia and its disorders, therapeutic importance of aspartic acid salts; outline of an experimental and clinical study, *Presse Med*, 66, 2125, 1958

464 Laborit, H., Magnier, R., Coirault, R., Thiebault, J., Guiot, G., Niaussat, P., Weber, B., Jouany, J. M., and Baron, C., The place of certain salts of DL-aspartic acid in the mechanisms of preservation of activity in reaction to the environment: summary of an experimental and clinical study, *Presse Med*, 66, 1307, 1958.

465. Rosen, H., Blumenthal, A., and Agersborg, H. P. K., Effects of potassium and magnesium salts of aspartic acid on metabolic exhaustion, *J Pharm Sci*, 51, 592, 1962.

466. Kendrich, Z. V., Tangsakul, S., Goldfarb, A., and Mole, P. A., Potassium aspartate treatment: effects on blood ammonia, urea and exercise to exhaustion, *Med Sci Sports*, 8, 70, 1976.

467. Matoush, L. O., Consolazio, C. F., Nelson, R. A., Isaac, G. J., and Torres, J. B., Effects of aspartic acid salts (Mg and K) on swimming performance of rats and dogs, *J Appl Physiol*, 19, 262, 1964

468. de Hann, A., van Doorn, J. E., and Westra, H. G., Effects of potassium and magnesium aspartate on muscle metabolism and force development during intensive static exercise, *Int J Sports Med*, 6, 44, 1985.

469. Nakahara, M., Yamada, S., Sakahashi, H., Nakanishi, Y., Tokita, T., and Yoshihars, T., Die Effekte von Kalium- und Magnesium-Asparaginat auf die zelluläre Erschöpfung der Skelettmuskulatur und Mechanismus, *Arzneim Forsch*, 14, 1191, 1964

470. Nakahara, M., Yoshihara, T., Tokita, T., Nakanishi, Y., Sakahashi, H., and Shibata, N., Difference in action between D- and L-potassium and magnesium aspartates, *Arzneim Forsch*, 16, 1491, 1966

471. Kruse, C. A., Treatment of fatigue with aspartic acid salts, *Northwest Med*, 60, 597, 1961

472. Shaw, D. L., Chesney, M. A., Tullis, I. F., and Agersborg, M. P. K., Management of fatigue: a physiological approach, *Am J Med Sci*, 243, 758, 1962.

473. Council on Drugs, A.M A., Potassium and magnesium aspartate (Spartase), *JAMA*, 183, 362, 1963

474. Fallis, N., Wilson, W. R., Tetreault, L. L., and Lasagna, L., Effect of potassium and magnesium aspartate on athletic performance, *JAMA*, 185, 129, 1963.

475. Consolazio, C. F., Nelson, R. A., Matoush, L. O., and Isaac, G. J., Effects of aspartic acid salts (Mg and K) on physical performance of men, *J Appl Physiol*, 19, 257, 1964

476. Ahlborg, B., Ekelund, L. G., and Nilsson, C. G., Effect of potassium-magnesium aspartate on the capacity for prolonged exercise in man. *Acta Physiol Scand*, 74, 238, 1968

477. Gupta, J. S. and Srivastava, K. K., Effect of potassium-magnesium aspartate on endurance work in man *Ind J Exp Biol*, 11, 392, 1973

478. Von Franz, I. W. and Chintanaseri, C., Über die Wirkung des Kalium-Magnesium-Aspartates auf die Ausdauerleistung unter besonderer Berücksichtigung des Aspartates, *Sportarzt Sportmed*, 28, 37, 1977

479. Nagle, F. J., Balke, B., Ganslen, R. V., and Davis, A. W., The mitigation of physical fatigue with "Spartase", *U S Civil Aeromed Res Inst*, 1, 1963

480. Wesson, M., McNaughton, L, Davies, P., and Tristram, S., Effects of oral administration of aspartic acid salts on the endurance capacity of trained athletes, *Res Q Exer Sport*, 59, 234, 1988

481. Hagen, R. D., Upton, S. J., Duncan, J. J., Cummings, J. M., and Gettman, L. R., Absence of effect of potassium-magnesium aspartate on physiologic response to prolonged work in aerobically trained man. *Int J Sports Med*, 3, 177, 1982

482. Maughan, R. J. and Sadler, D. J. M., The effects of oral administration of salts of aspartic acid on the metabolic response to prolonged exhausting exercise in man, *Int J Sports Med*, 4, 119, 1983

483. Gulewitch, V. S. and Krimberg, R., Zur Kenntnis der Extraktionsstoffe der Muskeln 2 Mitteilung über das Carnitin, *Hoppe-Seyler Z. Physiol Chem*, 45, 326, 1905

484. Fritz, I. B., The metabolic consequences of the effects of carnitine on long-chain fatty acid oxidation, in *Cellular Compartmentalization and Control of Fatty Acid Oxidation*, Gran, F C, Ed., Academic Press, New York, 1968, 39.

485. Engel, A. G. and Angelini, C., Carnitine deficiency of human skeletal muscle with associated lipid storage myopathy: a new syndrome, *Science*, 179, 899, 1973

486. Siliprandi, N., Carnitine and physical exercise, in *Biochemical Aspects of Physical Exercise*, Benzi, G, Packer, L, and Siliprandi, N, Eds., Elsevier, Amsterdam, 1986, 197

487. Rebouche, C. J. and Paulson, D. J., Carnitine metabolism and function in humans, *Annu Rev Nutr*, 6, 41, 1986

488. Borum, P. R., Carnitine, *Annu Rev Nutr*, 3, 233, 1983.

489. Cerretelli, P. and Marconi, C., L-Carnitine supplementation in humans The effects on physical performance, *Int J Sports Med*, 11(1), 1, 1990.

490. Lennon, D. L. F., Stratmen, F. W., Shrago, E., Nagle, F. J., Madden, M., Hanson, P., and Carter, A. L., Effects of acute moderate-intensity exercise on carnitine metabolism in men and women, *J Appl Physiol*, 55, 489, 1983.

491. Carlin, J. I., Reddan, W. G., Sanjak, M., and Hodach, R., Carnitine metabolism during prolonged exercise and recovery in humans, *J Appl Physiol*, 61, 1275, 1986.

492   Cooper, M. B., Forte, C. A., and Jones, D. A., Citrate interference with the determination of acetylcarnitine: a method for its elimination, *Clin Chim Acta*, 159, 291, 1986.

493   Marconi, C., Sassi, G., Carpinelli, A., and Cerretelli, P., Effects of L-carnitine loading on the aerobic and anaerobic performance of endurance athletes, *Eur J Appl Physiol* , 54, 131, 1985.

494   Deleted in proof.

495   Deleted in proof

496   Costill, D. L., Fink, W. J., Getchell, L. H., Ivy, J. L., and Witzmann, F. A., Lipid metabolism in skeletal muscle of endurance-trained males and females, *J Appl Physiol* , 47, 787, 1979

497   Dragan, G. J., Vasiliu, A., Georgescsu, E., and Dumas, I., Studies concerning chronic and acute effects of L-carnitine on some biological parameters in elite athletes, *Rev Roum Morphol Embryol Physiol Physiol* , 24, 23, 1987

498   Deleted in proof

499   Greig, C., Finch, K. M., Jones, D. A., Cooper, M., Sargeant, A. J., and Forte, C. A., The effect of oral supplementation with L-carnitine on maximum and submaximum exercise capacity, *Eur J Appl Physiol* , 56, 457, 1987

500   Dal Negro, R., Pomari, G., Zoccatelli, O., and Turco, P., Changes in physical performance of untrained volunteers: effects of L-carnitine, *Clin Trials J* , 23, 242, 1986.

501   Angelini, C., Vergani, L., Costa, L., Martinuzzi, A., Dunner, E., Marescotti, C., and Nosadini, R., Use of carnitine in exercise physiology, *Adv Clin Enzymol* , 4, 103, 1986

502   Cooper, M. B., Jones, D. A., Edwards, R. H. T., Corbucci, G. C., Montanari, G., and Trevisani, C., The effect of marathon running on carnitine metabolism and on some aspects of muscle mitochondrial activities and antioxidant mechanisms, *J Sports Sci* , 4, 79, 1986

503   Soop, M., Bjorkman, O., Cederblad, G., Hagenfeldt, H., and Wahren, J., Influence of carnitine supplementation on muscle substrate and carnitine metabolism during exercise, *Eur J Appl Physiol* , 64, 2394, 1988

504   Askew, E. W., Hecker, A. L., and Wise, W. R., Dietary carnitine and adipose tissue turnover rate in exercised trained rats *J Nutr* , 107, 132, 1977.

505   Askew, E. W., Dohm, G. L., Weiser, P. C., Huston, R. L., and Doub, W. H., Supplemental dietary carnitine and lipid metabolism in exercising rats, *Nutr Metab* , 24, 32, 1980

506   Negrao, C. E., Metabolic consequences of D- and L- Carnitine Administration in Chronically Trained and Untrained Rats. Ph.D. thesis, University of Wisconsin, Madison, 1986

507.   Otto, R. M., Shores, K. V. M., and Perez, H. R., The effect of L-Carnitine supplementation on endurance exercise, *Med Sci Sports Exer* , 19, S68, 1987

508   Shores, K. V., Otto, R. M., Wygand, J. W., and Perez, H. R., Effect of L-carnitine supplementation on maximal oxygen consumption and free fatty acid serum levels, *Med Sci Sports Exer* , 19, S68, 1987

509   Cereda, G. and Scolari, M., Effect of an energy stimulator on the performance of a group of young people: evaluation of a videogame test, *Acta Vitaminol Enzymol* , 6, 63, 1984

510   Dal Negro, R., Pomari, G., Zoccatelli, O., and Turco, P., L-Carnitine and rehabilitative physiokinesitherapy: metabolic and ventilatory response in chronic respiratory insufficiency, *Int J Clin. Pharmacol Ther Toxicol* , 24, 453, 1986.

511   Dal Negro, R., Turco, P., Pomari, G., and De Conti, F., Effects of L-carnitine on physical performance in chronic respiratory insufficiency. *Int J Clin Pharmacol Ther Toxicol* , 26, 269, 1988.

512.   Kosolcharoen, P., Nappi, J., Peducci, P., Shug, A., Patel, A., Filipek, T., and Thomsen, J. H., Improved exercise tolerance after administration of L-carnitine *Curr Ther Res* , 30, 753, 1981

513 Kamikawa, T., Suzuki, Y., Kobayashi, A., Hayashi, H., Masumura, Y., Nishihara, K., Abe, M., and Yamazaki, N., Effects of L-carnitine on exercise tolerance in patients with stable angina pectoris, *Jpn Heart J*, 25, 587, 1984.

514. Cherchi, A., Lai, C., Angelino, F., Trucco, G., Caponnetto, S., Mereto, P. E., Rosolen, G., Manzoli, U., Schiavoni, G., Reale, J. A., Romeo, F., Rizzon, P., Sorgente, L., Strano, A., Novo, S., and Immordino, R., Effects of L-carnitine on exercise tolerance in chronic stable angina: a multicenter, double-blind, randomized, placebo controlled cross-over study, *Int J. Clin Pharmacol Ther Toxicol*, 23, 569,1985.

515 Brevetti, G., Chiariello, M., Ferulano, G., Policicchio, A., Nevola, E., Rossinin, A., Attisano, R., Ambrosio, G., Siliprandi, M., and Angelini, C., Increases in walking distance in patients with peripheral vascular disease treated with L-carnitine: a double-blind, cross-over study, *Circulation*, 77, 767, 1988

516 Canale, C., Terrachini, V., Biagini, A., Vallebons, A., Masperone, M. A., Valice, S., and Castellano, A., Bicycle ergometer and echocardiographic study in healthy subjects and patients with angina pectoris after administration of L-carnitine: semiautomatic computerized analysis of M-mode tracing, *Int J Clin Pharmacol Ther Toxicol*, 26, 221, 1988.

517 DeGrandis, D., Mezzina, C., Fiaschi, A., Pinelli, P., Bazzato, G., and Morachiello, M., Myasthenia (muscle weakness) due to DL-carnitine treatment, *J Neurol Sci*, 46, 365, 1980

518 Bazzato, G., Coli, U., Landini, S., Mezzina, C., and Ciman, M., Myasthenia-like (muscle weakness) syndrome DL- but not L-carnitine, *Lancet*, 1, 1209, 1981.

519 Ernster, L. and Nelson, B., Functions of coenzyme Q, in *Biomedical and Clinical Aspects of Coenyme Q*, Vol 3, Folkers, K and Yamamura, Y, Eds., Elsevier, Amsterdam, 1981, 159

520 Folkers, K. and Yamamura, Y., Eds., *Biomedical and Clinical Aspects of Coenzyme Q*, Elsevier, Amsterdam, 1977

521 Yamamura, Y., Folkers, K., and Ito, Y., Eds., *Biomedical and Clinical Aspects of Coenzyme Q*, Vol. 2, Elsevier, Amsterdam, 1980.

522 Folkers, K. and Yamamura, Y., Eds., *Biomedical and Clinical Aspects of Coenzyme Q*, Vol 3, Elsevier, Amsterdam, 1981.

523 Folkers, K. and Yamamura, Y., Eds., *Biomedical and Clinical Aspects of Coenzyme Q*, Vol 4, Elsevier Amsterdam, 1984.

524 Beyer, R. E., Morales-Corral, P. G., Ramp, B. J., Kreitman, K. R., Falzon, M. J., Rhee, Y. S., Kuhn, T. W., Stein, M., Rosenwasser, M. J., and Cartwright, K. J., Elevation of tissue coenzyme Q (ubiquinone) and cytochrome c concentrations by endurance exercise in the rat, *Arch Biochem Biophys*, 234, 323, 1984

525 Shimomura, Y., Suzuki, M., Sugiyama, S., Hanaki, Y., and Ozawa, T., Protective effect of coenzyme Q_{10} on exercise-induced muscular injury, *Biochem Biophys Res Commun*, 176(1), 349, 1991

526 Leibovitz, B., Hu, M.-L., and Tappel, A. L., Dietary supplements of vitamin E, β-carotene, coenzyme Q_{10} and selenium protect tissues against lipid peroxidation in rat tissue slices, *J Nutr*, 120, 97, 1990

527 Awata, N., Ishiyama, T., Harada, H., Sawamura, A., Ogura, K., Tanimoto, T., Azuma, J., Hasegawa, H., Morita, Y., and Yamamura, Y., The effect of coenzyme Q_{10} on ischemic heart disease evaluated by dynamic exercise test, in *Biomedical and Clinical Aspects of Coenzyme Q*, Vol 2, Yamamura, Y., Folker, K., and Ito, Y., Eds, Elsevier, Amsterdam, 1980, 247

528 Hiasa, Y., Ishida, T., Maeda, T., Iwano, K., Aihara, T., and Mori, H., Effects of coenzyme Q_{10} on exercise tolerance in patients with stable angina pectoris, in *Biomedical and Clinical Aspects of Coenzyme Q*, Vol. 4, Folkers, K and Yamamura, Y, Eds, Elsevier, Amsterdam, 1984, 291.

529. **Vanfraechem, J. H. P., Picalusa, C., and Folkers, K.,** Effects of CoQ$_{10}$ on physical performance and recovery in myocardial failure, in *Biomedical and Clinical Aspects of Coenzyme Q*, Vol 5, Folkers, K. and Yamamura, Y., Eds , Elsevier, Amsterdam, 1986, 371

530. **Motomiya, T., Iyeki, K., Watanabe, K., Tokuyasu, Y., Sakurada, H., Ejiri, N., and Nanba, K.,** Elevated beta thromboglobulin in peripheral venous blood of patients with exercise-induced myocardial ischemia and its prevention with coenzyme Q$_{10}$, in *Biomedical and Clinical Aspects of Coenzyme Q*, Vol 5, Folkers, K and Yamamura, Y., Eds , Elsevier, Amsterdam, 1986, 379.

531 **Schardt, F., Welzel, D., Schiess, W., and Toda, K.,** Effect of coenzyme Q$_{10}$ on ischaemia-induced ST-segment depression: a double-blind, placebo-controlled crossover study, in *Biomedical and Clinical Aspects of Coenzyme Q*, Vol. 5, Folkers, K and Yamamura, Y., Eds., Elsevier, Amsterdam, 1986, 385

532 **Yamazaki, M., Kamikawa, T., Kobayashi, A., and Yamashita, T.,** Effects of coenzyme Q$_{10}$ on exercise tolerance in stable angina: a double-blind, randomized, placebo-controlled crossover trial, in *Biomedical and Clinical Aspects of Coenzyme Q*, Vol 5, Folkers, K and Yamamura, Y , Eds , Elsevier, Amsterdam, 1986, 395

533 **Vanfrechem, J. and Folkers, K.,** Coenzyme Q$_{10}$ and physical performance, in *Biomedical and Clinical Aspects of Coenzyme Q*, Vol 3, Folkers, K. and Yamamura, Y , Eds., Elsevier, Amsterdam, 1981, 235

534 **Zuliani, U., Bonetti, A., Campana, M., and Cerioli, G.,** The influence of ubiquinone (CoQ$_{10}$) on the metabolic response to work, *J Sports Med* , 29(1), 57, 1989.

535 **McGilvery, R. W., Ed.,** *Biochemistry: A Functional Approach*, 2nd ed., W. B. Saunders, Philadelphia, 1979, 361.

536 **Crim, M. C., Calloway, D. H., and Margen, S.,** Creatine metabolism in men: creatine pool size and turnover in relation to creatine intake, *J Nutr* , 106, 371, 1976

537 **Chanutin, A.,** The fate of creatine when administered to man, *J Biol Chem* , 67, 29, 1926

538 **Rose, W. C., Ellis, R. H., and Helming, O. C.,** The transformation of creatine into creatinine by the male and female organism *J Biol Chem* , 77, 171, 1928.

539. **Hyde, E.,** Creatine feeding and creatine-creatinine excretion in males and females of different age groups, *J Biol Chem* , 143, 301, 1942.

540 **Bleiler, R. E. and Schedl, H. P.,** Creatinine excretion: variability and relationships to diet and body size, *J Lab Clin Med* , 56, 945, 1962

541 **McCarty, M. F.,** Toward a "bio-energy supplement" — a prototype for functional orthomolecular supplementation, *Med Hypoth* , 7, 515, 1981.

542 **McGilvery, R. W., Ed.,** *Biochemistry A Functional Approach*, 2nd ed , W B Saunders, Philadelphia, 1979, 589

543 **Atzler, E. and Lehman, G.,** Die Wirkung von Lecithin auf Arbeitsstoffwechsel und Leistungsfähigkeit, *Arbeitsphysiol* , 9, 76, 1937.

544 **Staton, W.,** The influence of soya lecithin on muscular strength, *Res Q Am Health Phys Ed* , 22, 201, 1951

545 **Conaly, L. A., Wurtman, R. J., Blusztaijn, K., Coviella, I. L. G., Maher, T. J., and Evoniuk, G. E.,** Decreased plasma choline concentrations in marathon runners, *N Engl J Med* , 315, 892, 1986.

546 **Wurtman, R. J., Hirsch, M. J., and Growdon, J. H.,** Lecithin consumption raises serum free-choline levels *Lancet*, 2, 953, 1978.

547 **Hirsch, M. J., Growdon, J. H., and Wurtman, R. J.,** Relations between dietary choline or lecithin intake, serum choline levels, and various metabolic indices, *Metabolism*, 27, 953, 1978

548 **Wurtman, R. J.,** Nutrients that modify brain function, *Sci Am* , 246, 50, 1982.

549 **Chan, M. M.,** Choline and carnitine, in *Handbook of Vitamins: Nutritional, Biochemical and Clinical Aspects*, Machlin, L. J , Ed., Marcel Dekker, New York, 1984, 549.

550 **Krebs, E. T., Jr., Krebs, E. T., Sr., Harris, A. T., Bodman, J., Malin, R., and Beard, H. H.,** Pangamic acid sodium: a newly isolated crystalline water soluble factor — a preliminary report, *Rec Med* , 164, 18, 1951

551 Yakovlev, N. N., Leshkevich, L. G., and Kolomeitseva, B. I., The effect of pangamic acid (vitamin B15) on metabolism during physical exercise of varying duration, in *Vitamin B15 (Pangamic Acid) Properties, Functions and Uses*, Michlin, V. N., Ed., Science Publishing House (Naooka), Moscow, 1965, 182.

552 Karpuchina, Y. L., Oreshchenko, N. I., and Stolyarova, N. A., Effect of pangamic acid on biochemical changes in the blood of athletes during performance of exercises, in *Vitamin B15 (Pangamic Acid) Properties, Functions and Uses*, Michlin, V. N., Ed, Science Publishing House (Naooka), Moscow, 1965, 165

553 Cody, M. M., Substances without vitamin status, in *Handbook of Vitamins Nutritional, Biochemical and Clinical Aspects*, Machlin. L J., Ed., Marcel Dekker, New York, 1984, 571.

554 Beard, H. H. and Wofford, G., The effect of administration of synthetic vitamin $B_{15}H_8$ upon creatine formation in the rat. *Exp Med Surg*, 14 169, 1956

555 Gray, M. E. and Titlow, L. W., B_{15}: myth or miracle?, *Phys Sportsmed*, 10, 107, 1982.

556 Pipes, T. V., The effects of pangamic acid on performance in trained athletes, *Med Sci Sports Exer*, 12, 98, 1980

557 Kemp, G. L., A clinical study and evaluation of pangamic acid, *J Am Osteopath Assoc*, 58, 714, 1959

558 Gannon, J. R. and Kendall, R. V., A clinical evaluation of N,N-dimethylglycine (DGM) and diisopropylammonium dichloroacetate (DIPA) on the performance of racing grey-hounds, *Canine Pract*, 9, 23, 1982

559 Levine, S. B., Myhre, G. D., Smith, G. L., Burns, J. G., and Erb, B., Effect of a nutritional supplement containing N,N-dimethylglycine (DMG) on the racing standard-bred, *Equine Pract*, 4, 31, 1982

560 Dohm, G. L., Debnath, S., and Frisell, W. R., Effects of commercial preparations of pangamic acid (B_{15}) on exercised rats, *Biochem Med*, 28, 77, 1982.

561 Girandola, R. N., Wiswell, R. A., and Bulbulian, R., Effects of pangamic acid (B-15) ingestion on metabolic response to exercise, *Med Sci. Sports Exer*, 12, 98, 1980

562 Girondola, R. N., Wiswell, R. A., and Bulbulian, R., Effects of pangamic acid (B-15) ingestion on metabolic response to exercise, *Biochem Med*, 24, 218, 1980

563 Black, D. G. and Suec, A. A., Effects of calcium pangamate on aerobic endurance parameters A double-blind study, *Med. Sci Sports Exer*, 13, 93, 1981

564 Gray, M. E. and Titlow, L. W., The effect of pangamic acid on maximal treadmill performance, *Med Sci Sports Exer*, 14, 424, 1982.

565 Harpaz, M., Otto, R. M., and Smith, T. K., The effect of N_1N_1-dimethylglycine ingestion upon aerobic performance, *Med Sci Sports Exer*, 17, 287, 1985.

566 Bishop, P. A., Smith, J. F., and Young, B., Effects of N,N-dimethylglycine on physiological response and performance in trained runners, *J Sports Med Phys Fit*, 27, 53, 1987.

567 Friedman, M. A., Reaction of sodium nitrite with dimethlyglycine produces nitrososarcosine, *Bull Environ Cont Toxicol*, 13, 226, 1975

568. Colman, N., Herbert, V., Gardner, A., and Gelernt, M., Mutagenicity of dimethylglycine when mixed wih nitrite: possible significance in human use of pangamates, *Proc Soc Exp Biol Med*, 164, 9, 1980.

569 Shephard, S. E., Schlatter, C., and Lutz, W. K., Assessment of the risk of formation of carcinogenic N-nitroso compounds from dietary precursors in the stomach. *Food Chem Toxicol*, 25, 91, 1987

570 Kendall, R. V., Submitted for publication

571. McGilvery, R. W., *Biochemistry A Functional Approach*, 2nd ed., W. B. Saunders, Philadelphia, 1979, 644

572 de Verdier, C.-H. and Westman, M., Intravenous infusion of inosine in man: effect of erythrocyte 2,3-diphosphoglycerate concentration and on blood oxygen affinity, *Scand J Clin Lab Invest*, 32, 205, 1973

573 Akerblom, O., de Verdier, C.-H., Garby, L., and Hogman, C., Restoration of defective oxygen transport function of stored red blood cells by addition of inosine, *Scand J Clin Lab Invest*, 21, 245, 1968

574. **Lachieze-Rey, E.,** Experimentation de l'inosine en pathologie geriatrique, *Lyon Med*, 222, 83, 1969
575. **Linquette, M., Fossati, P., Luez, G., and Lefebvre, J.,** Experimentation clinique de l'inosine au cours des affections cardiovasculaires et en réanimation chirurgicale, *Lille Med*, 12, 265, 1967.
576. **Fox, I. H. and Kelley, W. N.,** The role of adenosine and 2'-deoxyadenosine in mammalian cells, *Annu. Rev Biochem.*, 47, 655, 1978.
577. **Colgan, M.,** Inosine, *Muscle Fitness*, 49, 94, 1988.
578. **McCord, J. M. and Fridovich, I.,** Superoxide dismutase. An enzymic function for erythrocuprein (hemocuprein), *J. Biol Chem.*, 244, 6049, 1969
579. **Brooke, M. H., Choksi, R., and Kaiser, K. K.,** Inosine monophosphate production is proportional to muscle force in vitro, *Neurology*, 36, 288, 1986.
580. **Kurtz, T. W., Kabra, P. M., Booth, B. E., Al-Bander, H. A., Portale, A. A., Serena, B. G., Tsai, H. C., and Morris, R. C.,** Liquid-chromatographic measurements of inosine, hypoxanthine, and xanthine in studies of fructose-induced degradation of adenine nucleotides in human and rats, *Clin Chem.*, 32, 782, 1986
581. **Halliwell, B. and Gutteridge, J. M. C.,** Eds., *Free Radicals in Biology and Medicine*, Clarendon Press, Oxford, 1985, 107.
582. **Roy, R. S. and McCord, J. M.,** Superoxide and ischemia: conversion of xanthine dehydrogenase to xanthine oxidase, in *Oxy-Radicals and Their Scavenger Systems*, Greenwald, R A. and Cohen, G, Eds., Elsevier, Amsterdam, 1983.
583. **Katz, A., Broberg, S., and Sahlin, K.,** Beta-adrenoreceptor blockade results in excessive formation of IMP and ammonia during exercise in humans, *Med Sci Sports Exer*, 20, S62, 1988
584. **Knochel, J. P., Dotin, L. N., and Hamberger, R. J.,** Heat stress, exercise, and muscle injury: effects on urate metabolism and renal function, *Ann Int Med*, 81, 321, 1974.
585. **Sjödin, B. and Westing, Y. H.,** Changes in plasma concentration of hypoxanthine and uric acid in man with short-distance running at various intensities, *Int J Sports Med*, 11(6), 493, 1990
586. **Lowenstein, J. M.,** The purine nucleotide cycle revised, *Int J Sports Med*, 11(Suppl. 2), S37, 1990
587. **McGilvery, R. W.,** Ed., *Biochemistry: A Functional Approach*, 2nd ed., W. B. Saunders, Philadelphia, 1979, 655.
588. **Berlin, R. D. and Hawkins, R. A.,** Secretion of purines by the small intestine: general characteristics, *Am. J Physiol.*, 215, 932, 1968
589. **Roll, P. M., Brown, G. B., DiCarlo, F. J., and Schultz, A. S.,** The metabolism of yeast nucleic acid in the rat, *J Biol Chem.*, 180, 333, 1968.
590. **de Verdier, C.-H., Garby, L., Hjelm, M., and Hogman, C.,** Adenine in blood preservation: posttransfusion viability and biochemical changes, *Transfusion*, 4, 331, 1964
591. **Schimert, G.,** Therapie und Prophylaxe der Koronarerkrankungen mit nukleosidhalten Wirkstoffen, *Med. Monatsschr.*, 25, 415, 1971
592. **Feiks, F. K.,** Zur Therapie des Myokardinfarktes, *Wien. Med Wochenschr*, 15, 338, 1960
593. **Lindblad, G., Jonsson, G., and Falk, J.,** Adenine toxicity: a three week intravenous study in dogs, *Acta Pharm Toxicol*, 32, 246, 1973
594. **Martin, P.,** Calcium et entrainement, *Schweiz Med Wochenschr*, 69, 125, 1939
595. **Greenleaf, J. E. and Brock, P. J.,** Na$^+$ and Ca2$^+$ ingestion: plasma volume-electrolyte distribution at rest and exercise, *J Appl. Physiol*, 48, 838, 1980.
596. **Greenleaf, J. E.,** Hyperthermia and exercise, in *Environmental Physiology III*, Vol. 20, Robertshaw, D., Ed., University Park Press, Baltimore, 1979, 157
597. **Avioli, L. V.,** Calcium and osteoporosis, *Annu Rev. Nutr*, 4, 471, 1984
598. **Dawson-Hughes, B.,** Osteoporosis and aging: gastrointestinal aspects, *J Am Coll Nutr*, 5, 393, 1986
599. **Brooks-Gunn, J., Warren, M. P., and Hamilton, L. H.,** The relation of eating problems and amenorrhea in ballet dancers, *Med Sci Sports Exer*, 19, 41, 1987.

600 Linnell, S. L., Stager, J. M., Blue, P. W., Oyster, N., and Robertshaw, D., Bone mineral content and menstrual regularity in female runners, *Med Sci Sports Exer*, 16, 343, 1984

601 Oyster, N., Morton, M., and Linnell, S., Physical activity and osteoporosis in postmenopausal women, *Med Sci Sports Exer*, 16, 44, 1984.

602. Smith, E. L., Jr., Reddan, W., and Smith, P. E., Physical activity and calcium modalities for bone mineral increase in aged women, *Med Sci Sports Exer*, 13, 60. 1981.

603. Smith, E. L., Jr., Smith, P. E., Ensign, C. J., and Shea, M. M., Bone involution decrease in exercising middle-aged women, *Calcif Tissue Int*, 36 (Suppl), S129, 1984.

604. Stillman, R. J., Lohman, T. G., Slaughter, M. H., and Massey, B. H., Physical activity and bone mineral content in women aged 30 to 85 years, *Med Sci. Sports Exer*, 18, 576, 1986

605 Lee, C. J., Lawler, G. S., and Johnson, G. H., Effects of supplementation of the diet with calcium and calcium-rich foods on bone density of elderly females with osteoporosis, *Am J Clin Nutr*, 34, 819, 1981.

606. Wolinsky, I. and Telang, S. D., Calcium metabolism and needs in the elderly, in *CRC Handbook of Nutrition in the Aged*, Watson. R R., Ed., CRC Press, Boca Raton, FL, 1985, 123.

607. Williams, M. H., The role of minerals in physical activity, in *Nutritional Aspects of Human Physical Performance*, 2nd ed, Charles C Thomas, Springfield, IL, 1985, 186

608 Bulbulian, R., Girandola, R. N., Wiswell, R. A., and Koyal, S. N., The effect of NH_4Cl induced chronic metabolic acidosis on work capacity in man, *Med Sci Sports Exer*, 13, 85, 1981.

609 Mautalen, C. A., Cabrejas, M. L., and Soto, R. J., Isotopic determination of intestinal calcium absorption in normal subjects, *Metabolism*, 18, 395, 1969

610 Liu, L., Borowski, G., and Rose, L. I., Hypomagnesemia in a tennis player, *Phys Sportsmed*, 11, 79, 1983

611 Casoni, I., Guglielmini, C., Graziano, L., Reali, M. G., Mazzotta, D., and Abbasciano, V., Changes of magnesium concentrations in endurance athletes, *Int J Sports Med*, 11(3), 234, 1990

612 Steinacker, J. M., Grünert-Fuchs, M., Steininger, K., and Wodick, R. E., Effects of long-time administration of magnesium on physical capacity, *Int J. Sports Med*, 8, 151, 1987

613. Risser, W. L. and Risser, J. M. H., Iron deficiency in adolescents and young adults, *Phys Sportsmed*, 18(12), 87, 1990.

614 Anderson, H. T. and Stavem, P., Iron deficiency and the acid-base variations of exercise, *Nutr Metab*, 14, 129, 1972

615 Davies, C. T. M. and van Haaren, J. P. M., Effect of treatment on physiological responses to exercise in East African industrial workers with iron deficiency anaemia, *Br J Ind Med*, 30, 335, 1973

616 Hermansen, L., Oxygen transport during exercise in human subjects, *Acta Physiol Scand Suppl*, 399, 9, 1973

617 Gardner, G. W., Edgerton, V. R., Barnard, R. J., and Bernauer, E. M., Cardiorespiratory, hematological and physical performance responses of anemic subjects to iron treatment *Am J Clin Nutr*, 28, 982, 1975

618 Edgerton, V. R., Gardner, G. W., Ohira, Y., Gunawarden, K. A., and Senewirante, B., Iron deficiency anaemia and its effect on worker productivity and activity patterns, *Br Med J*, 2, 1549, 1979.

619 Ohira, Y., Edgerton, V. R., Gardner, G. W., Senewirante, B., Barnard, R. J., and Simpson, D. R., Work capacity, heart rate and blood lactate responses to iron treatment, *Br J Haem*, 41, 365, 1979

620 Ohira, Y., Edgerton, V. R., Gardner, G. W., Senewirante, B., and Simpson, D. R., Blood gas content in iron deficient and anemic subjects before and after iron treatment, *Med Sci Sports Exer*, 14, 109, 1982

621 Nickerson, H. J. and Tripp, A. D., Iron deficiency in adolescent cross-country runners, *Phys Sportsmed*, 11, 60, 1983.

622. Hunding, A., Jordal, R., and Pauley, P. E., Runner's anemia and iron deficiency, *Acta Med. Scand*, 209, 315, 1981.

623 Nilson, K., Schoene, R. B., Robertson, H. T., Escourrou, P., and Smith, N. J., The effect of iron repletion on exercise-induced lactate production in minimally iron-deficient subjects, *Med Sci Sports Exer*, 13, 92, 1981.

624 Plowman, S. and McSwegin, P., The effects of iron supplementation on female cross-country runners, *J. Sports Med*, 21, 247, 1981.

625. Schoene, R. B., Nilson, K., Robertson, H. T., Excourrou, P., and Smith, N. J., The effect of iron repletion on exercise-induced lactate production in minimally iron-deficient subjects, *Clin Res*, 29, 452A, 1981

626 Schoene, R. B., Escourrou, P., Robertson, H. T., Nilson, K. L., Parsons, J. R., and Smith, N. J., Iron repletion decreases maximal exercise lactate concentrations in female athletes with minimal iron deficiency anemia, *J Lab Clin Med*, 102, 306, 1983.

627. Rowland, T. W., Diesroth, M. B., and Green, G. M., The effect of iron therapy on the exercise capacity of nonanemic iron-deficient adolescent runners, *Am J Dis Child*, 14, 165, 1988

628. Rowland, T. W., Deisroth, M., and Kelleher, J. F., The effect of iron therapy on the exercise capacity of non-anemic iron deficient female high school runners, *Med Sci Sports Exer*, 19, S20, 1987.

629 Risser, W. L., Lee, E. J., Poindexter, H. B. W., West, M. S., Pivarnik, J. M., Risser, J. M. J., and Hickson, J. F., Iron deficiency in female athletes: its prevalence and impact on performance, *Med Sci Sports Exer*, 20, 116, 1988.

630. Lamanca, J. and Haymes, E., Effects of dietary iron supplementation on endurance, *Med Sci Sports Exer.*, 21 (Suppl. 2), S77, 1989.

631 Barry, A., Cantwell, J. T., Doherty, F., Folan, J. C., Ingoldsby, M., Kevany, J. P., O'Brien, J. D., O'Conner, H., O'Shea, B., Ryan, B. A., and Vaughan, J., A nutritional study of Irish athletes, *Br J Sports Med*, 15, 99, 1981

632. Brotherhood, J., Brozovic, B., and Pugg, L. G., Haematological status of middle and long distance runners, *Clin Sci Mol. Med*, 48, 139, 1975.

633. Weswig, P. and Winkler, W., Iron supplementation and hematological data of competition swimmers, *J Sports Med*, 14, 112, 1974.

634 Cooter, G. R. and Mowbray, K., Effects of iron supplementation and activity on serum iron depletion and hemoglobin levels in female athletes, *Res Q*, 49, 114, 1978

635. Pate, R. R., Maguire, M., and Van Wyk, J., Dietary iron supplementation in women athletes, *Phys Sportsmed*, 7, 81, 1979

636. Hegenauer, J., Strause, L., Saltman, P., Dann, D., White, J., and Green, R., Transitory effects of moderate exercise are not influenced by iron supplementation, *Eur J Appl Physiol*, 52, 57, 1983.

637. Dressendorfer, R. H., Keen, C. L., Wade, C. E., Claybaugh, J. R., and Timmis, G. C., Development of runner's anemia during a 20-day road race: effect of iron supplements, *Int J Sports Med*, 12(3), 332, 1991.

638 Embden, G., Grafe, E., and Schmitz, E., Über Steigerung der Leistungsfähigkeit durch Phosphatzufuhr, *Z Physiol Chem*, 113, 67, 1921

639 Herxheimer, H., Zur Wirkung von primaren Natriumphosphate auf die korperliche leistungsfähigkeit, *Klin Wochenschr*, 1, 480, 1922.

640. Hingberg, K., Über den Einfluss von Phosphat auf den Sauerstoffverbrauch bei der Arbeit, *Z Exp Med*, 59, 262, 1928.

641. Poppelreuter, W., Zur Frage der Steigerung der industriellen Arbeistfähigkeit durch Recresalzufuhr, *Arbeitsphysiol.*, 2, 507, 1930.

642. Poppelreuter, W., Selbstbeobachtungen über die Wirkung jahrelanger Phosphatzufuhr, *Arbeitsphysiologie*, 3, 605, 1930.

643. Herxheimer, H., Zur Physiologie der maximalen Muskelarbeit in Sport, *Z Physik Ther*, 44, 55, 1933

644. Atzler, E., Bergmann, K., Graf, O., Kraut, H., Lehmann, G., and Szakall, A., Phosphat und Arbeit, *Arbeitsphysiologie*, 8, 621, 1935.

645 Szakall, A., Über den Phosphatstoffwechsel bei Muskelarbeit, *Arbeitsphysiologie*, 8, 316, 1935

646 Kaunitz, H. and Austria, G. F., Muscle fatigue (relations to permeability, mineral metabolism, lactate metabolism and use of oxygen by tissues), *Acta Med Philipp*, 1, 369, 1940

647 Ehrenberg, R., Über die Wirkung langerdauernder Phosphatzufuhr auf den Stoffwechsel in Ruhe und Arbeit, *Dtsch Med Wochenschr*, 73, 44, 1948.

648 Danilov, A., Korjakina, A., Kossovskaja, E., Krestownikoff, A., and Fomicov, A., Der Einfluss der Phosphat auf den Wasser und Salzumsatz bei Muskelarbeit, *Arbeitsphysiologie*, 8, 1, 1935.

649 Kogan, G. and Krestownikoff, A., Der Einfluss von Monophosphaten auf die hauttemperatur bei Muskelarbeit, *Arbeitsphysiologie*, 8, 24, 1935

650. Krestownikoff, A., Korjakina, A., Kossowskaja, E., Retelskaja, P., and Schirobokow, S., Die Wirkung von Monophosphaten auf das Blut und den Blutkreislauf bei Korperlicher Arbeit, *Arbeitsphysiologie*, 8, 13, 1935

651 Latmanisowa, L. W., Einwirkung der Phosphate auf die Änderungen der Muskelchronazxie bei Arbeit, *Arbeitsphysiologie*, 8, 147, 1935

652 Puni, A., Der Einfluss von Monophosphaten auf einige psychische und psychomotorische Prozesse Wahrend der Erholungspenode nach Muskelarbeit, *Arch Psychol*, 86, 459, 1932

653 Flynn, F. B., The so-called action of acid sodium phosphate in delaying the onset of fatigue, *U S Health Rep*, 41, 1463, 1929

654 Talbott, J. H., Folling, A., Henderson, L. J., Dill, D. B., Edwards, H. T., and Berggren, R. E. L., Studies in muscular activity; changes and adaptations in running, *J Biol Chem*, 78, 445, 1928.

655 Riabuschinsky, N. P., Einfluss der Darreichung von Phosphaten per os auf die Arbeitsfähigkeit und den Gaswechsel, *Z Exp Med*, 72, 20, 1930.

656 Rahm, K., Über die Wirkung des Recresals auf die körperliche und geistige Leistungsfähigkeit, *Arch Psychol*, 86, 459, 1932

657 Marbe, K., Über die vermeintliche Leistungssteigerung durch Recresol und Natrium Bicarbonicum, *Arch Exp Pathol Pharmakol*, 167, 404, 1932.

658 Sauser-Hall, P., L'emploi du C-Phos dans les troupes d'elite, *Schweiz Med Wochenschr*, 72, 197, 1942

659 Keller, W. D. and Kraut, H. A., Work and nutrition, *World Rev. Nutr Diet*, 3, 65, 1959

660 Cade, R., Conte, M., Zauner, C., Mars, D., Peterson, J., Lunne, D., Hommen, N., and Packer, D., Effects of phosphate loading on 2,3-diphosphoglycerate and maximal oxygen uptake, *Med Sci Sports Exer*, 16, 263, 1984

661 Duffy, D. J. and Conlee, R. K., Effects of phosphate loading on leg power and high intensity treadmill exercise, *Med. Sci Sports Exer*, 18, 674, 1986

662 Sapega, A. A., Sokolow, D. P., Graham, T. J., and Chance, B., Phosphorus nuclear magnetic resonance: a non-invasive technique for the study of muscle bioenergetics during exercise, *Med Sci Sports Exer*, 19, 410, 1987

663. Lane, H. W., Some trace elements related to physical activity: zinc, copper, selenium, chromium and iodine, in *Nutrition in Exercise and Sport*, Hickson, J F. and Wolinsky, I, Eds, CRC Press, Boca Raton, FL, 1989, 301.

664 Levander, O. A. and Burk, R. F., Selenium, in *Present Knowledge in Nutrition*, Brown, M L., Ed, International Life Sciences Institute — Nutrition Foundation, Washington, D C, 1990, 268.

665 Brady, P. S., Ku, P. K., and Ullrey, D. E., Lack of effect of selenium supplementation on the response of the equine erythrocyte glutathione system and plasma enzymes to exercise, *J Anim Sci*, 47, 492, 1978

666 Brady, P. S., Brady, L. J., and Ullrey, D. E., Selenium, vitamin E and the response to swimming stress in the rat, *J Nutr*, 109, 1103, 1979

667 Ono, K., Inui, K., Hasegawa, T., and Matsuki, N., The changes of antioxidative enzyme activities in equine erythrocytes following exercise, *Nippon Juigaku Zasshi*, 52(4), 759, 1990

668 Dragan, I., Dinu, V., Mohora, M., and Cristea, E., Studies regarding the antioxidant effects of selenium on top swimmers, *Rev Roum Physiol.*, 27(1), 15, 1990

669. Stoecker, B. J., Chromium, in *Present Knowledge in Nutrition*, Brown, M. L , Ed., International Life Sciences Institute — Nutrition Foundation, Washington, D C., 1990, 287.

670 Anderson, R. A. and Kozlovsky, A. S., Chromium intake, absorption and excretion of subjects consuming self selected diets, *Am J Clin Nutr.*, 41, 1177, 1985

671. Anderson, R. A., Polansky, M. M., Bryden, N. A., Roginski, E. E., Patterson, K. Y., and Reamen, D. C., Effect of exercise (running) on serum glucose, insulin, glucagon, and chromium excretion, *Diabetes*, 31, 212, 1982

672. Anderson, R. A., Polansky, M. M., and Bryden, N. A., Strenuous running: acute effects on chromium, copper, zinc, and selected clinical variables in urine and serum of male runners, *Biol Trace Element Res* , 6, 327, 1984

673 Anderson, R. A., Bryden, N. A., Polansky, M. M., and Deuster, P. A., Exercise effects on chromium excretion of trained and untrained men consuming a constant diet, *J Appl Physiol* , 64, 249, 1988.

674. Evans, G. W., The effect of chromium picolinate on insulin controlled parameters in humans, *Int J Biosoc Med Res* , 11, 163, 1989

675 Clarkson, P. M., Nutritional ergogenic aids: chromium, exercise, and muscle mass, *Int J Sports Nutr* , 1, 289, 1991

676 Frantz, A. G. and Rabkin, M. T., Effects of estrogen and sex differences on secretion of human growth hormone, *J Clin Endocrinol* , 25, 1470, 1965.

677. Knopf, R. F., Conn, J. W., Falans, S. S., Floyd, J. C., Guntsche, E. M., and Rull, J. A., Plasma growth hormone responses to intravenous administration of amino acids, *Clin Endocrinol* , 25, 1140, 1965

678 Merimee, T. J., Burgess, J. A., and Rabinowitz, D., Sex-determined variation in serum insulin and growth hormone response to amino acid stimulation, *J Clin Endocrinol* , 26, 791, 1966

679. Rabinowitz, D., Merimee, T. J., Burgess, J. A., and Riggs, L., Growth hormone and insulin release after arginine: indifference to hyperglycemia and epinephrine, *J Clin Endocrinol* , 26, 1170, 1966

680. Merimee, T. J., Rabinowitz, D., Riggs, L., Burgess, J. A., Rimoin, D. L., and McKusick, V. A., Plasma growth hormone after arginine infusion. Clinical experiences, *N Engl J Med.*, 276, 434, 1967.

681. Merimee, T. J. and Fineberg, S. E., Studies of the sex based variation of human growth hormone, *J Clin Endocrinol* , 33, 896, 1971

682. Gourmelen, M., Donnadieu, M., Schimpff, R. M., Lestradet, H., and Girard, F., Effect of ornithine monochloride on plasma HGH levels, *Ann Endocrinol.*, 33, 526, 1972

683 Rakoff, J. S., Siler, T. M., Sinha, Y. N., and Yen, S. S. C., Prolactin and growth hormone release in response to sequential stimulation by arginine and synthetic TRF, *J Clin Endocrinol* , 37, 641, 1973

684. Bratusch-Marrain, P. and Waldhausl, W., The influence of amino acids and somatostatin on prolactin and growth hormone release in man, *Acta Endocrinol* , 90, 403, 1979.

685 Siler, T. M., Van den Berg, G., Yen, S. S. C., Brazeau, P., Vale, W., and Guillemin, R., Inhibition of growth hormone release in humans by somatostatin, *J Clin Endocrinol* , 37, 632, 1973

686 Mochizuki, M., Morkawa, H., Kawaguchi, K., and Tojo, S., Growth hormone, prolactin and chorionic somatomammotropin in normal and molar pregnancy, *J Clin Endocrinol* , 43, 614, 1976.

687. Onishi, T., Itoh, K. F., Miyai, K., Izumi, K., Shima, K., and Kumahara, Y., Prolactin response to arginine in normal subjects and in patients with hyperthyroidism, *J Clin. Endocrinol* , 42, 148, 1976

688. **Penny, R., Blizzard, R. M., and Davis, T.,** Sequential arginine and insulin tolerance test on the same day, *J Clin Endocrinol*, 29, 1499, 1969

689. **Job, J. C., Sizonenko, P. C., and Balage, M.,** Interpretation statistique des epreuves de stimulation de la secretion d'hormone de croissance par l'insuline et l'argine, *Arch Franc Ped (Paris)*, 28, 505, 1971.

690. **Braverman, E. R. and Pfeiffer, C. C., Eds.,** Arginine and citrulline, in *The Healing Nutrients Within Facts, Findings and New Research on Amino Acids,* Keats Publishing, New Canaan, CT, 1986, 173

691. **Pearson, D. and Shaw, S., Eds.,** *Life Extension A Practical Scientific Approach,* Warner Books, New York, 1982, 192.

692 **Mathieni, G.,** Growth hormone secretion by arginine stimulus: the effect of both low doses and oral arginine, *Boll Soc It Sper Biol*, 56, 2254, 1980.

693. **Besset, L.,** Increase in sleep related growth hormone and prolactin secretion after chronic arginine aspartate administration, *Acta Endocrinol*, 99, 18, 1982

694 **Elsair, C.,** Effets de l'arginine, administrie par voie orale, *C R Soc Biol*, 179, 608, 1985

695. **Isidori, A., Lo Monaco, A., and Cappa, M.,** A study of growth hormone release in man after oral administration of amino acids, *Curr Med Res Opinion*, 7, 475, 1981

696 **McGilvery, R. W., Ed.,** *Biochemistry. A Functional Approach,* 2nd ed., W. B. Saunders, Philadelphia, 1979, 555.

697. **Bessman, S. P.,** Blood ammonia, *Adv Clin Chem*, 2, 135, 1959.

698 **Mutch, B. J. C. and Banister, E. W.,** Ammonia metabolism in exercise and fatigue: a review, *Med Sci Sports Exer*, 15, 41, 1983.

699. **Banister, E. W., Rajendra, W., and Mutch, B. J. C.,** Ammonia as an indicator of exercise stress: implications of recent findings to sports medicine, *Sports Med*, 2, 34, 1985

700. **Greenstein, J. P., Winitz, M., Gullino, P., and Birnbaum, S. M.,** The prevention of ammonia toxicity by L-arginine and related compounds, *Arch Biochem Biophys*, 59, 302, 1955

701. **Gullino, P., Winitz, M., Birnbaum, S. M., Cornfield, J., Otey, M. C., and Greenstein, J. P.,** Studies on the metabolism of amino acids and related compounds in vivo. 1 Toxicity of essential amino acids, individually and in mixtures, and the protective effect of L-arginine, *Arch Biochem Biophys*, 64, 319, 1956.

702 **Winitz, M., Gullino, P., Greenstein, J. P., and Birnbaum, S. M.,** Studies on the metabolism of amino acids and related compounds in vivo II. Effect of toxic doses of essential amino acids on blood sugar, liver glycogen and muscle glycogen levels, *Arch Biochem Biophys*, 64, 333, 1956.

703 **Greenstein, J. P., Winitz, M., Gullino, P., Birnbaum, S. M., and Otey, M. C.,** Studies on the metabolism of amino acids and related compounds in vivo. III. Prevention of ammonia toxicity by arginine and related compounds, *Arch Biochem Biophys*, 64, 342, 1956

704. **du Ruisseau, J. P., Greenstein, J. P., Winitz, M., and Birnbaum, S. M.,** Studies on the metabolism of amino acids and related compounds in vivo IV. Blood ammonia and urea levels following intraperitoneal administration of amino acids and ammonium acetate, and the effect of arginine thereon, *Arch Biochem Biophys.*, 64, 355, 1956

705 **Winitz, M., du Ruisseau, J. P., Otey, M. C., Birnbaum, S. M., and Greenstein, J. P.,** Studies on the metabolism of amino acids and related compounds in vivo V Effects of combined administration of nonprotective compounds and subprotective levels of L-arginine HCL on ammonia toxicity in rats, *Arch Biochem Biophys*, 64, 368, 1956

706 **Harper, H. A., Najarian, J. S., and Silen, W.,** Effect of intravenously administered amino acids on blood ammonia, *Proc Soc Exp Biol Med*, 92, 558, 1956

707 **Najarian, J. S. and Harper, H. A.,** Comparative effect of arginine and monosodium glutamate on blood ammonia, *Proc Soc Exp Biol Med*, 92 560, 1956

708 **Greenstein, J. P., du Ruisseau, J. P., Winitz, M., and Birnbaum, S. M.,** Studies on the metabolism of amino acids and related compounds in vivo VII Ammonia toxicity in partially hepatectomized rats and the effect of L-arginine thereon, *Arch Biochem Biophys*, 71, 458, 1957

709   Fahey, J. L., Toxicity and blood ammonia rise resulting from intravenous amino acid administration in man: the protective effect of L-arginine, *J Clin Invest*, 36, 1647, 1957.

710. Gullino, P., Winitz, M., Birnbaum, S. M., Otey, M. C., Cornfield, J., and Greenstein, J. P., Toxicity of essential amino acid mixtures with special reference to the protective effect of L-arginine, *Arch Biochem Biophys*, 58 255, 1958.

711   Bessman, S. P., The reduction of blood ammonia levels by certain amino acids, *J Clin Invest*, 35, 69, 1959.

712   Najarian, J. S. and Harper, H. A., A clinical study of the effect of arginine on blood ammonia, *Am J Med*, 21, 832, 1956.

713   Elam, R. P., Morphological changes in adult males from resistance exercise and amino acid supplementation, *J Sports Med*, 28, 35, 1988.

714   Barnes, R. H., Labadan, B. A., Siyamoglu, R., and Bradfield, R. B., Effects of exercise and administration of aspartic acid on blood ammonia in the rat, *Am J Physiol*, 207, 1242, 1964.

715   Salvatore, F., Scoppa, P., and Cozzolino, D., Protective effect of ornithine and aspartic acid in chronic carbon tetrachloride intoxication, *Clin Chim Acta*, 4, 728, 1959

716   Salvatore, F. and Bocchini, V., Prevention of ammonia toxicity by amino acids concerned in the biosynthesis of urea, *Nature*, 191, 705, 1961.

717   Cutinelli, L., Sorrentino, L., Tramonti, C., Salvatore, F., and Cedrangelo, F., Protection by ornithine-aspartate of the effects of physical exercise, *Arzneim Forsch*, 20, 1064, 1970.

718   Braverman, E. R. and Pfeiffer, C. C., Aspartic acid — asparagine, in *The Healing Nutrients Within Facts, Findings and New Research on Amino Acids*, Keats Publishing, New Canaan, CT, 1986, 225

719   Liljenquist, J. E., Lacy, W. W., Chiasson, J. L., and Rabinowitz, D., Regulation of alanine and branched chain amino acid metabolism in intact man, in *Clinical Nutrition Update Amino Acids*, Greene, H L., Holliday, M A., and Munro, H N, Eds, AMA, Chicago, 1979, 22.

720   Walser, M. and Williamson, J. R., Eds., *Metabolism and Clinical Implications of Branched Chain Amino and Ketoacids*, Elsevier, New York, 1981

721   Harper, A. E., Miller, R. H., and Block, K. P., Branched-chain amino acid metabolism, *Annu Rev Nutr*, 4, 409, 1984.

722. Braverman, E. R. and Pfeiffer, C. C., Leucine, isoleucine and valine, in *The Healing Nutrients Within Facts, Findings and New Research on Amino Acids*, Keats Publishing, New Canaan, CT, 1986, 269

723   Albanese, A. A., Orto, L. A., and Zavattaro, N., Nutrition and metabolic effects of physical exercise, *Nutr. Rep Int*, 3, 165, 1971.

724. Rocha, D. M., Faloona, G. R., and Unger, R. H., Glucagon stimulating activity of 20 amino acids in dogs, *J Clin Invest*, 51, 2346, 1972

725   Munro, H. N., Metabolism and functions of amino acids in man — overview and synthesis, in *Amino Acids Metabolism and Medical Applications*, Blackburn, G L, Grant, J P., and Young, V. R, Eds., John Wright/PSG, Boston, 1983, 1.

726   Walshe, J. M., The effect of glutamic acid on the coma of hepatic failure, *Lancet*, 1, 1075, 1953.

727   McDermott, W. V., Adams, R. D., and Riddell, A. G., Treatment of hepatic coma with L-glutamic acid, *N Engl J Med*, 253, 1093, 1955

728   Bessman, S. P., Shear, S., and Fitzgerald, J., Effect of arginine and glutamate on removal of ammonia from blood in normal and cirrhotic patients, *N Engl J Med*, 256, 941, 1957.

729   Brodan, V., Kuhn, E., Pechar, J., Placer, Z., and Slabochova, Z., Effects of sodium glutamate infusion on ammonia formation during intense physical exercise in man, *Nutr Rep. Int*, 9, 223, 1974

730   Braverman, E. R. and Pfeiffer, C. C., Glutamic acid, GABA and glutamine, in *The Healing Nutrients Within Facts, Findings and New Research on Amino Acids*, Keats Publishing, New Canaan, CT, 1986, 205.

731. **Brand, E., Harris, M. M., Sandberg, W., and Ringer, A. I.,** Studies on the origin of creatine, *Am J Physiol*, 90, 296, 1929.

732 **Boothby, W. M.,** Myasthenia gravis; preliminary report on effect of treatment with glycine, *Proc Mayo Clin*, 7, 557, 1932

733 **Boothby, W. M.,** Myasthenia gravis; second report on the effect of treatment with glycine, *Proc Mayo Clin*, 7, 737, 1932.

734 **Thomas, K., Milhorat, A. T., and Techner, F.,** Untersuchungen über die Herkunft des Kreatins. Ein Beitrag zur Behandlung progressiver Muskeltrophien mit Glykokoll, *Z Physiol Chem*, 204, 93, 1932.

735 **Milhorat, A. T.,** Über dier Behandlung der progressiven Muskeldystrophie und Ähnlicher Muskelerkrankungen mit Glykokoll, *Dtsch Arch Klin Med*, 174, 487, 1933.

736 **Kostakow, S. and Slauck, A.,** Die Glykokollbehandlung der progressiven Muskeldystrophie. Zugleich ein Beitrag zur Herkunft des Kreatins, *Arch Klin Med*, 175, 25, 1933

737 **Boothby, W. M.,** The clinical effect of glycine in progressive muscular dystrophy, in simple fatigability and on normal controls, *Proc Staff Meet, Mayo Clin*, 9, 600, 1934

738 **Cuthbertson, D. P. and MacLachlan, T. K.,** Treatment of muscular dystrophy with glycine, *Q J Med*, 3, 411, 1934.

739 **Reinhold, J. G., Clark, J. H., Kingsley, G. R., Custer, R. P., and McConnell, J. W.,** Effects of glycine (glycocoll) in muscular dystrophy, with special references to changes in structure and composition of voluntary muscle, *JAMA*, 102, 261, 1934

740. **Tripoli, C. J. and Beard, H. H.,** Muscular dystrophy and atrophy; clinical and biochemical results following oral administration of amino acids, *Arch Int Med*, 53, 435, 1934

741 **Armstrong, C. N. and Herbert, F. K.,** Glycine treatment of progressive muscular dystrophy, *Newcastle Med J*, 15, 71, 1934

742. **Boothby, W. M.,** Treatment of progressive muscular dystrophy with glycine, *J Pediatr*, 6, 725, 1935

743. **Nevin, S.,** A critical review· primary diseases ot voluntary muscles, *J Neurol Psychiatr*, 1, 120, 1938

744. **Reinhold, J. G. and Kingsley, G. R.,** The chemical composition of voluntary muscle in muscle disease; a comparison of progressive muscular dystrophy with other diseases together with a study of effects of glycine and creatine therapy, *J Clin Invest*, 17, 377, 1938.

745. **Beard, H. H., Ed.,** *Creatine and Creatinine Metabolism*, Brooklyn Chemical Publishers, Brooklyn, NY, 1943

746 **Hench, P. S.,** A consideration of muscular pain and fatigue with a note on glycine: preliminary comment, *Proc Staff Meet, Mayo Clin*, 9, 603, 1934.

747 **McGuire, S.,** Glycine in the treatment of chronic fatigability, *Int J Med Surg*, 47, 459, 1934.

748 **Wilder, R. M.,** Discussion of reports by Drs Boothby and Hench, *Proc Staff Meet, Mayo Clin*, 9, 606, 1934

749 **Chaikelis, A. S.,** The effect of glycocoll (glycine) ingestion upon the growth, strength and creatinine-creatine excretion in man, *Am J Physiol*, 132, 578, 1941

750. **Maison, G. L.,** Failure of gelatin or aminoacetic acid to increase the work ability, *JAMA*, 115, 1439, 1940

751 **Horvath, S. M., Knehr, C. A., and Dill, D. B.,** The influence of glycine on muscular strength, *Am J Physiol*, 134, 469, 1941

752. **King, E. Q., McCaleb, L. B., Kennedy, H. F., and Klumpp, T. G.,** Failure of aminoacetic acid to increase the work capacity of human subjects, *JAMA*, 118, 594, 1942

753 **Hilsendager, D. and Karpovich, P. V.,** Ergogenic effect of glycine and niacin separately and in combination, *Res Q*, 35, 389, 1964

754 **Braverman, E. R. and Pfeiffer, C. C.,** Glycine, in *The Healing Nutrients Within Facts, Findings and New Research on Amino Acids*, Keats Publishing, New Canaan, CT, 1986, 237

755. **Quick, A. J.,** The conjunction of benzoic acid in man, *J Biol Chem*, 92, 283, 1980

756. **Kasai, K., Kobayashi, M., and Shimoda, S.,** Stimulatory effect of glycine on human growth hormone secretion, *Metabolism*, 27, 201, 1978
757. **Kasai, K., Suzuki, H., Nakamura, T., Shiina, H., and Shimoda, S.,** Glycine stimulates growth hormone in man, *Acta Endocrinol*, 93, 283, 1980.
758. **Lassarre, C., Girard, F., Durand, J., and Raynaud, J.,** Kinetics of human growth hormone during submaximal exercise, *J Appl Physiol*, 37, 826, 1974.
759 **Shephard, R. J. and Sidney, K. H.,** Effects of physical exercise on plasma growth hormone and cortisol levels in human subjects, *Exer Sport Sci Rev*, 3, 1, 1975
760. **Galbo, H., Richter, E. A., Hilsted, J., Holst, J. J., Christensen, N. J., and Henriksson, J.,** Hormonal regulation during prolonged exercise, *Ann N Y Acad Sci*, 301, 72, 1977.
761 **Sutton, J. R.,** Effect of acute hypoxia on the hormonal response to exercise, *J Appl Physiol*, 42, 587, 1977
762 **Karagiorgos, A., Garcia, J. F., and Brooks, G. A.,** Growth hormone response to continuous and intermittent exercise, *Med. Sci Sports Exer*, 11, 302, 1979
763 **Kinderman, W., Schnabel, A., Schmitt, W. M., Biro, G., Cassens, J., and Weber, F.,** Catecholamines, growth hormone, cortisol, insulin, and sex hormones in anaerobic and aerobic exercise, *Eur J Appl Physiol.*, 49, 389, 1982
764 **Barwich, D., Rettenmeier, A., Weicker, H., and Schwarz, W.,** Stress hormones in the serum of athletes after successive exertions, in *Current Topics in Sports Medicine*, Bachl, N, Prokop, L., and Suckert, R., Eds., Urban and Schwarzenberg, Baltimore, MD, 1984, 420.
765 **Wolf, W, Schmid, P., Schwaberger, G., and Pessenhofer, H.,** The behavior of cortisol, insulin, HGH and glucagon serum levels under the effect of short- and longtime physical exertion in athletes, in *Current Topics in Sports Medicine*, Bachl, N., Prokop, L, and Suckert, R, Eds., Urban and Schwarzenberg, Baltimore, MD, 1984, 433
766 **McCollum, R. H.,** The Effect of L-lysine and a Vitamin Compound upon the Physical Performance of Subpar College Men, Ed D. thesis, University of Oregon, Eugene, 1960
767 **Donnadieu, M., Combourieu, M., and Schimpff, R. M.,** Comparison de différentes épreuves de stimulation utilisées pour l'étude de la fonction somatotrope chez l'infant, *Pathol Biol*, 19, 293, 1971.
768 **Evian-Brion, D., Donnadieu, M., Roger, M., and Job, J. C.,** Simultaneous study of somatotrophic and corticotrophic pituitary secretions during ornithine infusion test, *Clin Endocrinol*, 17, 119, 1982.
769 **Braverman, E. R. and Pfeiffer, C. C.,** Eds., Ornithine, in *The Healing Nutrients Within Facts, Findings and New Research on Amino Acids*, Keats Publishing, New Canaan, CT, 1986, 186
770 **Bucci, L. R., Hickson, J. F., Pivarnik, J. M., Wolinsky, I., McMahon, J. C., and Turner, S. D.,** Ornithine ingestion and growth hormone release in bodybuilders, *Nutr Res*, 10, 239, 1990.
771 **Bucci, L. R., Klenda, B.A., Hickson, J. F., and Wolinksy, I.,** Ornithine levels in human serum after oral dosing measured by a colorimetric assay, *J Nutr Biochem*, 2, 363, 1991.
772. **Hickson, J. F., Bucci, L. R., Wolinsky, I., Pivarnik, J. M., Turner, S., and McMahon, J. C.,** Effect of oral ornithine amino acid supplementation on serum insulin levels, *J Appl Sport Sci Res*, 4(3), 108, 1990.
773 **Bucci, L. R., Hickson, J. F., Wolinsky, I., and Pivarnik, J. M.,** Ornithine supplementation and insulin release in bodybuilders, *Int J Sports Nutr*, 2, 287, 1992.
774 **Cynober, L., Coudray-Lucas, C., de Bandt, J. P., Guechot, J., Aussel, C., Salvucci, M., and Gibodeau, J.,** Action of ornithine-α-ketoglutarate, ornithine hydrochloride, and calcium α-ketoglutarate on plasma amino acid and hormonal patterns in healthy subjects, *J Am Coll Nutr*, 9, 2, 1990.
775 **Oratz, M., Rothschild, M. A., Schrieber, S. S., Burks, A., Mongelli, J., and Matarese, B.,** The role of the urea cycle and polyamines in albumin synthesis, *Hepatology*, 3, 567, 1983

776 Tabor, H. and Tabor, C. W., Biosynthesis and metabolism of 1,4-diamino butane, spermidine, spermine and related amines, *Adv Enzymol.*, 36, 203, 1972.

777 Lescoat, G., Desvergne, B., Loreal, O., Pasdeloup, N., Deugnier, Y., Bourel, M., and Brissot, P., Modulation of albumin secretion by ornithine alpha-ketoglutarate in adult rat hepatocyte cultures and a human hepatoma cell line (HepG₂), *Ann. Nutr Metab*, 33, 252, 1989

778 Cynober, L., Vauboudelle, M., Dore, A., and Gibodeau, J., Kinetics and metabolic effects of orally administered ornithin-α-ketoglutarate in healthy subjects fed with a standardized regimen, *Am J Clin Nutr*, 39, 514, 1984.

779 Cynober, L., Ornithine α-ketoglutarate in nutritional support, *Nutrition*, 7(5), 1, 1991.

780 Silk, D. B. A. and Payne-James, J. J., Novel substrates and nutritional support: possible role of ornithine α-ketoglutarate, *Proc Nutr Soc*, 49, 381, 1990.

781 Muller, E. E., Brambilla, F., Cavagnini, F., Peracchi, M., and Panerai, A., Slight effect of L-tryptophan on growth hormone release in normal human subjects, *J Clin Endocrinol Metab.*, 39, 1, 1974.

782 Woolf, P. D. and Lee, L., Effect of the serotonin precursor, tryptophan, on pituitary hormone secretion, *J Clin Endocrinol Metab*, 45, 123, 1977.

783 Fraser, W. M., Tucker, H. S., Grubb, S. R., Wigand, J. P., and Blackard, W. G., Effect of L-tryptophan on growth hormone and prolactin release in normal volunteers and patients with secretory pituitary tumors, *Horm Metab Res*, 11, 149, 1979.

784 Glass, A. R., Schaaf, M., and Dimond, R. C., Absent growth hormone response to L-tryptophan in acromegaly, *J Clin Endocrinol. Metab*, 48, 664, 1979.

785 Koulu, M. and Lammintausta, R., Effect of methionin on L-tryptophan and apomorphine-stimulated growth hormone secretion in man, *J Clin Endocrinol Metab*, 49, 70, 1979.

786 Hartmann, E., L-tryptophan: a rational hypnotic with clinical potential, *Am. J Psychiatr*, 134, 366, 1977.

787 Sandyk, R., Consroe, P. F., and Iacono, R. P., L-tryptophan in drug-induced movement disorders with insomnia, *N. Engl J Med*, 314, 1237, 1986.

788 Furst, P., Guarnieri, G., and Hultman, E., The effect of the administration of L-tryptophan on synthesis of urea and gluconeogenesis in man, *Scand J Clin Lab Invest*, 27, 183, 1971.

789. Segura, R. and Ventura, J. L., Effect of L-tryptophan supplementation on exercise performance, *Int J Sports Med*, 9, 301, 1988.

790. Slutsker, L., Eosinophilia-Myalgia Syndrome associated with exposure to tryptophan from a single manufacturer, *JAMA*, 264(2), 213, 1990

791. Belongia, R., An investigation of the cause of the Eosinophilia-Myalgia Syndrome associated with tryptophan use, *N Engl J Med*, 323(6), 357, 1990

792. Jaffe, R., Eosinophilia Myalgia Syndrome secondary to contaminated tryptophan — clinical experience, *J Nutr Med*, 2, 195, 1991

793. Aldhous, P., Yellow light on L-tryptophan, *Nature*, 353, 490, 1991.

794 Williams, M. H., Ed., Ergogenic foods, in *Nutritional Aspects of Human Physical and Athletic Performance*, 2nd ed, Charles C Thomas, Springfield, IL, 1985, 312.

795 Cockerill, D. L. and Bucci, L. R., Increases in muscle girth and decreases in body fat associated with a nutritional supplement program, *Chiroprac Sports Med*, 1, 73, 1987.

796 Ushakov, A., Effect of vitamin and amino acid supplements on human physical performance during heavy mental and physical work, *Aviat Space Environ Med*, 49, 1184, 1978

797 Barnett, D. W. and Conlee, R. K., The effects of a commercial dietary supplement on human performance, *Am J Clin Nutr*, 40, 586, 1984.

798 Weight, L. M., Myburgh, K. H., and Noakes, T. D., Vitamin and mineral supplementation: effect on the running performance of trained athletes, *Am J Clin Nutr*, 47, 192, 1988.

799 Anderson, T., Moffit, J., Fahrenbach, B., and Dunford, M., The ergogenic effect of Enerzymes, *J Appl Sport Sci Res*, 4(3), 111, 1990

800. **Keul, J. and Haralambie, G.,** Effect of a multivitamin-electrolyte-granulate on blood circulation and metabolism in protracted effort, *Schweiz Z Sportmed* , 22, 164, 1974

801. **Swislocki, A. L. M., Chen, Y.-D., Goley, A., Chang, M.-O., and Reaven, G. M.,** Insulin suppression of plasma free fatty acid concentration in normal individuals or patients with Type II (non insulin dependent) diabetes, *Diabetologia*, 30, 622, 1987

802. **Galbo, H.,** Endocrinology and metabolism in exercise, *Int J Sports Med* , 2, 125, 1981

803. **Unger, R. H. and Lefebvre, P. J.,** *Glucagon: Molecular Physiology, Clinical and Therapeutic Implications*, Pergamon Press, Oxford, UK, 1972.

804 **Hunter, W. M. and Sukkar, M. Y.,** Changes in plasma insulin levels during muscular exercise, *J Physiol* , 196, 110, 1968

805 **Bottger, I., Schlein, E. M., Faloona, G. R., Knochel, J. R., and Unger, R. H.,** The effect of exercise on glucagon secretion, *J Clin Endocrinol* , 35, 117, 1972.

806. **Felig, P., Wahren, J., Hendler, R., and Ahlber, G.,** Plasma glucagon levels in exercising man, *N Engl J Med* , 287, 184, 1972.

807. **Williams, M. H.,** Drug foods — alcohol and caffeine, in *Nutritional Aspects of Human Physical and Athletic Performance,* 2nd ed , Charles C Thomas, Springfield, IL, 1985, 272

808 **Graham, D. M.,** Caffeine — its identity, dietary sources, intake and biological effects, *Nutr Rev* , 36, 97, 1978

809. **Slavin, J. L. and Joensen, D. J.,** Caffeine and sports performance, *Phys Sportsmed* , 13, 191, 1985

810 **Van Handel, P.,** Caffeine, in *Ergogenic Aids in Sports,* Williams, M. H , Ed., Human Kinetics Publishers, Champaign, IL, 1983, 128.

811 **Williams, M. H., Ed.,** Caffeine, in *Drugs and Athletic Performance,* Charles C Thomas, Springfield, IL, 1974, 48

812. **Ganslen, R. V., Balke, B., Nagle, F., and Phillips, E.,** Effects of some tranquilizing analeptic and vasodilating drugs on physical work capacity and orthostatic tolerance, *Aerospace Med* , 35, 630, 1964.

813 **Margaria, R., Aghemo, P., and Rovelli, E.,** The effect of some drugs on the maximal capacity of athletic performance in men, *Int Z Angew Physiol* , 20, 281, 1964

814 **Lovingood, B. W., Blyth, C. S., Peacock, W. H., and Lindsay, R. B.,** Effects of d-amphetamine sulfate, caffeine, and high temperature on human performance, *Res Q* . 38, 64, 1967

815 **Perkins, R. and Williams, M. H.,** Effect of caffeine upon maximal muscular endurance of females, *Med Sci Sports,* 7, 221, 1975

816 **Costill, D. L., Dalsky, G. P., and Fink, W. J.,** Effects of caffeine ingestion on metabolism and exercise performance, *Med Sci Sports Exer* , 10, 155, 1978

817. **Temples, T. and Haymes, E.,** The effects of caffeine on substrate metabolic and body temperature responses during exercise in a cold and neutral environment, *Med Sci Sports Exer* , 15, 157, 1983

818 **Essig, D., Costill, D. L., and Van Handel, P. J.,** Effects of caffeine ingestion on utilization of muscle glycogen and lipid during leg ergometer cycling, *Int J Sports Med* , 1, 86, 1980

819 **Ben-Ezra, V. and Vaccaro, P.,** The influence of caffeine on the anaerobic threshold of competitively trained cyclists, *Med Sci Sports Exer* , 14, 176, 1982.

820 **Berglund, B. and Hemmingson, P.,** Effects of caffeine ingestion on exercise performance at low and high altitudes in cross-country skiers, *Int J Sports Med* , 3, 234, 1982

821 **Temples, T. and Haymes, E.,** The effects of caffeine on substrates in a cold and neutral environment, *Med Sci Sports Exer* , 14, 176, 1982

822 **Toner, M. M., Kirkendall, D. T., Delio, D. J., Chase, J. M., Cleary, P. A., and Fox, E. L.,** Metabolic and cardiovascular responses to exercise with caffeine, *Ergonomics.* 25, 1175, 1982.

823 **Cadarette, B. S., Levine, L., Berube, C. L., Posner, B. M., and Evans, W. J.,** Effects of varied dosages of caffeine on endurance exercise to fatigue, in *Biochemistry of Exercise,* Knuttgen, H G., Vogel, J. A., and Poortmans, J , Eds., Human Kinetics Publishers. Champaign, IL, 1983, 871

824   Knapik, J. J., Jones, B. J., Toner, M. M., Daniels, W. L., and Evans, W. J., Influence of caffeine on serum substrate changes during running in trained and untrained individuals, in *Biochemistry of Exercise*, Knuttgen, H G., Vogel, J A., and Poortmans, J., Eds., Human Kinetics Publishers, Champaign, IL, 1983, 514

825   Powers, S., Byrd, R., Tulley, R., and Callender, T., Effects of caffeine ingestion on metabolism and performance during graded exercise, *Eur J. Appl Physiol*, 40, 301, 1983.

826   Butts, N. K. and Crowell, D., Effect of caffeine ingestion on cardiorespiratory endurance in men and women, *Res Q*, 56, 301, 1985.

827. Casal, D. C. and Leon, A. S., Failure of caffeine to affect substrate utilization during prolonged running, *Med Sci Sports Exer*, 17, 174, 1985.

828   Gaesser, G. A. and Rich, R. G., Influence of caffeine on blood lactate response during incremental exercise, *Int J Sports Med*, 6, 207, 1985

829   Fisher, S. M., McMurray, R. G., Berry, M., Mar, M. H., and Forsythe, W. A., Influence of caffeine on exercise performance in habitual caffeine users, *Int J Sports Med*, 7, 276, 1986.

830   Axelrod, J. and Reichenthal, J., The fate of caffeine in man and a method for its estimation in biological material, *J Pharmacol Exp Ther*, 107, 519, 1953

831. Eddy, N. B. and Downs, A. W., Tolerance and cross-tolerance in the human subject to the diuretic effect of caffeine, theobromine and theophylline, *J Pharmacol Exp Ther*, 33, 167, 1928

832   Colton, T., Gosswlin, R. E., and Smith, R. P., The tolerance of coffee drinkers to caffeine, *Clin Pharmacol Ther*, 9, 31, 1968

833   Goldstein, A., Kaizer, S., and Whitby, O., Psychotropic effects of caffeine in man. IV. Quantitative and qualitative differences associated with habituation to coffee, *Clin Pharmacol Ther*, 10, 489, 1969

834   Robertson, D., Wade, D., Workman, R., Wousley, R. L., and Oats, J. A., Tolerance to the humoral and hemodynamic effects of caffeine in man, *J Clin Invest*, 67, 1111, 1981.

835   Weir, J., Noakes, T. D., Myburgh, K., and Adams, B., A high carbohydrate diet negates the metabolic effects of caffeine during exercise, *Med Sci Sports Exer*, 19, 100, 1987.

836   Brust, M., Fatigue and caffeine effects in fast-twitch and slow-twitch muscles of the mouse, *Pfluegers Arch*, 367, 189, 1976

837   Giles, D. and Maclaren, D., Effects of caffeine and glucose ingestion on metabolic and respiratory functions during prolonged exercise, *J Sports Sci*, 2, 35, 1984

838   Powers, S. K., Dodd, S., Woodyard, J., and Mangum, M., Caffeine alters ventilatory and gas exchange kinetics during exercise, *Med Sci. Sports Exer*, 18, 101, 1986.

839   Erickson, M. A., Schwarzkopf, R. J., and McKenzie, R. D., Effects of caffeine, fructose, and glucose ingestion on muscle glycogen utilization during exercise, *Med Sci Sports Exer*, 19, 579, 1987

840   McNaughton, L., Two levels of caffeine ingestion on blood lactate and free fatty acid responses during incremental exercise, *Res Q Exer Sport*, 58, 255, 1987

841   Jacobson, B. H. and Edwards, S. W., Caffeine and neuromuscular performance, *Med Sci Sports Exer*, 19, S44, 1987.

842   Mamimori, G. H., Hetzler, R. K., Somani, S. M., Knowlton, R. G., and Perkins, R. M., The interactive effects of obesity and route of administration on caffeine metabolism during prolonged submaximal exercise, *Med Sci Sports Exer*, 19, S44, 1987.

843   Northey, D. R., Russell, C. A., Alway, S. A., Green, H. J., and Hughson, R. L., Propanolol and caffeine effects on metabolism in prolonged exercise, *Med Sci Sports Exer*, 19, S33, 1987

844   Hsieh, S., Bilanin, J., Haberman, K., and Doubt, T., Effects of caffeine and cold on exercise metabolism, *Med Sci Sports Exer*, 20, S84, 1988

845   Hetzler, R. K., Knowlton, R. G., Somani, S. M., Brown, D. D., and Perkins, R. M., Influence of paraxanthine on plasma free fatty acid concentrations, *Med Sci Sports Exer*, 19, S75, 1987.

846   Tommerdahl, A., Noble, B., and Wilkinson, J., Effect of caffeine on free fatty acid mobilization and respiratory quotient during prolonged running, *Med Sci Sports Exer*, 19, S44, 1987

847. Titlow, L. W., Ishee, J. H., and Riggs, C. E., Failure of caffeine to affect exercise metabolism, *Med Sci Sports Exer*, 19, S44, 1987

848 Wilcox, A. R., Effects of exercise on body fat levels of the rat, *Int. J Sports Med*, 6, 322, 1985

849 Wilcox, A. R., The effects of caffeine and exercise on body weight, fat-pad weight, and fat-cell size, *Med Sci Sports Exer*, 14, 317, 1982.

850 Delbeke, F. T. and Debackere, M., Caffeine: use and abuse in sports, *Int J. Sports Med*, 5, 179, 1984

851 Stillner, V., Popkin, M. K., and Pierce, C. M., Caffeine induced delirium during prolonged competitive stress, *Am J Psychiatr*, 135, 855, 1978

852 Bruni, O. J., *Gamma Oryzanol — The Facts*, Claudell Publishing, Houston, TX, 1989.

853 Ishihama, A., Hamatsu, Y., and Ito, T., On the effects of gamma oryzanol upon anterior lobe of rat pituitary, *Yokohama Med Bull*, 17(5), 183, 1966.

854 Yamauchi, J., Takahara, J., Uneki, T., Yakushiji, W., Nakashima, Y., Miyoshi, M., and Ofuji, T., The effect of gamma oryzanol on rat pituitary hormone secretion, *Folia Endocrinol Jpn*, 56(8), 1130, 1980.

855. Ieiri, T., Kase, N., Hashigami, Y., Kobori, H., Nakamura, T., and Shimoda, S., The effects of gamma oryzanol on the hypothalamo-pituitary axis in the rat, *Folia Endocrinol Jpn*, 58(10), 1350, 1982

856. Gorewit, R. C., Pituitary and thyroid hormone responses of heifers after ferulic acid administration, *J Dairy Sci*, 66, 624, 1983.

857. Yagi, K. and Ohishi, N., Action of ferulic acid and its derivatives as antioxidants, *J Nutr Sci Vitaminol*, 25, 127, 1979

858. Tajima, K., Sakamoto, M., Okada, K., Mukai, K., Ishizu, K., Mori, H., and Sakurai, H., Reaction of biological phenolic antioxidants with superoxide generated by cytochrome P450 model system, *Biochem Biophys. Res Commun.*, 115(3), 1002, 1983

859. Bors, W., Michel, C., ErbenRuss, M., Kreileder, B., Tait, D., and Saran, M., Rate constants of sparingly water-soluble phenolic antioxidants with hydroxyl radicals, in *Oxygen Radicals in Chemistry and Biology*, Bors, W., Saran, M., and Tait, D., Eds., Walter de Gruyter, Berlin, 1984, 95.

860. Yin, Z. Z., Wang, J. P., and Xu, L. N., Effect of sodium ferulate on malondialdehyde production from the platelets of rats, *Acta Pharmacol Sin.*, 7(4), 336, 1986.

861. Ohta, S., Furukawa, M., and Shinoda, M., Chemical protectors against radiation. 23 Radioprotective activities of ferulic acid and its related compounds, *Yakugaku Zasshi*, 104(7), 793, 1984.

862. Ishihara, M., Effect of gamma oryzanol on serum lipid peroxide level and clinical symptoms of patients with climacteric disturbances, *Asia-Oceania J Obstet Gynaecol*, 10(3), 317, 1984

863. Bucci, L. R., A natural magic bullet?, *Flex*, April, 25, 1989

864. Bucci, L. R., Blackman, G., Defoyd, W., Kaufmann, R., Mandel-Tayes, C., Sparks, W. S., Stiles, J. C., and Hickson, J. F., Effect of ferulate on strength and body composition of weightlifters, *J Appl Sport Sci. Res*, 4(3), 104, 1990.

865. Bonner, B., Warren, B., and Bucci, L., Influence of ferulate supplementation on postexercise stress hormone levels after repeated exercise stress, *J Appl Sport Sci Res*, 4(3), 110, 1990

866 Ray, G. B., Johnson, J. R., and Taylor, M. M., Effect of gelatine on muscular fatigue, *Proc Soc Exp Biol Med*, 40, 157, 1939

867. Kaczmarek, R. M., Effect of gelatin on the work output of male athletes and non-athletes and girl subjects, *Res Q*, 11, 4, 1940.

868. Kaczmarek, R. M., Relative influence of exercise, gelatine and sham feeding on work output, heart and pulse rates, *Med Rec*, 153, 383, 1941.

869 Dill, D. B., Knehr, C. A., Robinson, S., and Neufeld, W., Gelatin and muscular fatigue, cited in Milhorat, A. T., *Dtsch Arch Klin Med*, 174, 487, 1933.

870. **Hellebrandt, F. A., Rork, R., and Brogdon, E.,** Effect of gelatin on power of women to perform maximal anaerobic work, *Proc Soc Exp Biol Med ,* 43, 629, 1940
871. **Hellebrandt, F. A. and Karpovich, P. V.,** Fitness, fatigue and recuperation, *War Med ,* 1, 745, 1941
872. **Karpovich, P. V. and Pestrecov, K.,** Effect of gelatin upon muscular work in man, *Am J Physiol ,* 134, 300, 1941.
873. **Pryor, G. B. and Knapp, M. L.,** Effect of gelatin feeding on strength and weight according to body build, *Lancet,* 61, 484, 1941
874. **Robinson, S. and Harmon, P. M.,** The effects of training and of gelatin upon certain factors which limit muscular work, *Am J Physiol ,* 13, 161, 1941.
875 **Gissal, F. W. and Hall, L. K.,** Analysis of urinary hydroxyproline levels and delayed muscle soreness resulting from high and low intensity step testing under gelatin-free and gelatin-load dietary regimens, *Med Sci Sports Exer ,* 15, 165, 1983.
876. **Prockop, D. J. and Sjverdsma, A.,** Significance of urinary hydroxyproline in man, *J Clin Invest ,* 40, 843, 1961.
877 **Anon.,** Ginseng: western myth or eastern promise?, *IPU Rev ,* 9, 69, 1984
878 **Avakian, E. V. and Evonuk, E.,** Effect of Panax ginseng extract on tissue glycogen and adrenal cholesterol depletion dunng prolonged exercise, *Planta Med ,* 36, 43, 1979
879 **Avakian, E. V. and Sugimoto, B. R.,** Effect of Panax ginseng extract on blood energy substrates dunng exercise, *Fed Proc ,* 39, 287, 1980
880 **Wang, B., Cui, J., Liu, A., and Wu, S.,** Studies on the anti-fatigue effect of the saponins of stems and leaves of Panax ginseng (SSLG), *J Tradit Chin Med ,* 3, 89, 1983.
881 **Avakian, E. V., Sugimoto, R. B., Taguchi, S., and Horvath, S. M.,** Effect of Panax ginseng extract on energy metabolism during exercise in rats, *Planta Med.,* 50, 151, 1984.
882 **Samira, M. M. H., Attia, M. A., Allam, M., and Elwan, O.,** Effect of standardized ginseng extract G115 on the metabolism and electrical activity of the rabbit's brain, *J Int Med Res ,* 13, 342, 1985
883 **Takagi, K., Saito, H., and Tsuchiya, M.,** Effect of Panax ginseng root on spontaneous movement and exercise in mice, *Jpn J Pharmacol ,* 24, 41, 1974
884 **Saito, H., Yoshida, Y., and Takagi, K.,** Effect of Panax ginseng root on exhaustive exercise in mice, *Jpn J Pharmacol ,* 24, 119, 1974.
885 **Saito, H. and Bao, T.,** Effects of red ginseng, vitamins and their preparations. I Effect of forced exercise on mice, *Yakuri to Chiryo,* 12, 1453, 1984
886 **Yamamoto, M., Takeuchi, N., Kumagai, A., and Yamamura, Y.,** Stimulatory effect of Panax ginseng principles on DNA, RNA, protein and lipid synthesis in rat bone marrow, *Arzneim Forsch ,* 27, 1169, 1977
887 **Forgo, I. and Kirchdorfer, A.,** Ginseng stiegert die Körperliche Leistung, *Arztlich Praxis,* 33, 1784, 1981
888. **Knapik, J. J., Wright, J. E., Welch, M. J., Patton, J. F., Suek, L. L., Mello, R. P., Rock, P. B., and Teves, M. A.,** The influence of Panax ginseng on indices of substrate utilization during repeated, exhaustive exercise in man, *Fed Proc ,* 42, 336, 1983
889 **Teves, M. A., Wright, J. E., Welch, M. J., Patton, J. F., Mello, R. P., Rock, P. B., Knapik, J. J., Vogel, J. A., and der Marderosian, A.,** Effects of ginseng on repeated bouts of exhaustive exercise, *Med. Sci Sports Exer ,* 15, 162, 1983
890 **McNaughton, L., Egan, G., and Caelli, G.,** A comparison of Chinese and Russian ginseng as ergogenic aids to improve various facets of physical fitness, *Int Clin Nutr Rev ,* 9(1), 32, 1989
891. **Pieralisi, G.,** Effects of a standardized ginseng extract combined with dimethylaminoethanol bitartrate, vitamins, minerals, and trace elements on physical performance during exercise, *Clin Ther ,* 13(3), 373, 1991.
892 **Anon.,** The root of ginseng's power, *Health Store News,* Feb/Mar, 24, 1987

893 **Huang, H. M., Johanning, G. I., and O'Dell, B. L.,** Phenolic acid content of food plants and possible nutritional implications, *J. Agric Food Chem*, 34(1), 48, 1986

894. **Cureton, T. K. and Pohndorf, R. H.,** Influence of wheat germ oil as a dietary supplement in a program of conditioning exercises with middle-aged subjects, *Res Q*, 26, 391, 1955

895. **Cureton, T. K.,** Improvements in physical fitness associated with a course of U S. Navy underwater trainees, with and without dietary supplements, *Res Q*, 34, 440, 1963

896. **Brozek, B.,** Soviet studies on nutrition and higher nervous activity, *Ann N Y Acad Sci*, 93, 665, 1963

897 **Saint-John, M. and McNaughton, L.,** Octacosanol ingestion and its effects on metabolic responses to submaximal cycle ergometry, reaction time and chest and grip strength, *Int Clin Nutr Rev.*, 6, 81, 1986.

898 **Poiletman, R. and Miller, H.,** The influence of wheat germ oil on the electrocardiographic T waves of the highly trained athlete, *J Sports Med*, 8, 26, 1968

899. **Ershoff, B. H. and Levin, E.,** Beneficial effect of an unidentified factor in wheat germ oil on the swimming performance of guinea pigs, *Fed Proc*, *Fed Am Soc Exp Biol*, 14, 341, 1955.

900 **Consolazio, C. F., Matoush, L. O., Nelson, R. A., Isaac, G. J., and Hursh, L. M.,** Effect of octacosanol, wheat germ oil, and vitamin E on performance of swimming rats, *J Appl Physiol*, 19, 265, 1964.

901 **Entenman, C., Coughlin, J., and Ackerman, P. D.,** Substrate utilization and maximum swimming ability in rats and guinea pigs fed wheat germ oil, *Proc. Soc Exp Biol Med*, 141, 43, 1972

902. **Snider, S. R.,** Octacosanol in Parkinsonism, *Ann Neurol*, 16, 723, 1984

903. **Norris, F. H., Denys, E. H., and Fallat, R. J.,** Trial of octacosanol in amyotrophic lateral sclerosis, *Neurology*, 36, 1263, 1986.

904. **Rabinovitch, R., Gibson, W. C., and MacEachern, D.,** Neuromuscular disorders amenable to wheat germ oil therapy, *J Neurol Neurosurg Psychiatr*, 14, 95, 1951.

905 **Milhorat, A. T., Toscani, V., and Bartels, W. E.,** Effect of wheat germ oil on creatinuria in dermatomyositis and progressive muscular dystrophy, *Proc Soc Exp Biol Med*, 58, 40, 1945

906 **Jethon, Z., Szczurek, A. L., and Put, A.,** Effects of additional supply of minerals and vitamins on physical work capacity in strength sports, in *Symposium for Sportsmen*, Cernelle, A. B, Ed, Helsingborg, Sweden, 1972, 173

907 **Steben, R. E., Wells, J. C., and Harless, I. L.,** The effect of bee pollen tablets on the improvement of certain blood factors and performance of male collegiate swimmers, *J Natl Athletic Trainers Assoc*, 11, 124, 1976

908 **Durbisay, J.,** A new approach to the natural treatment of protein malnutrition, Results of a double-blind clinical trial, *Gaz Med. de France*, 40, 7674, 1973.

909 **Anon.,** Polbax® — nature's own antioxidant, Holomed International, Malmo, Sweden, 1991

910 **Steben, R. E. and Boudreaux, P.,** The effects of pollen and protein extracts on selected factors and performance of athletes, *J Sports Med*, 18, 221, 1978.

911 **Maughan, R. J. and Evans, S. P.,** Effects of pollen extract upon adolescent swimmers, *Br J Sports Med*, 16, 142, 1982

912 **Chandler, J. V. and Hawkins, J. D.,** The effect of bee pollen on physiological performance, *Med Sci Sports Exer*, 17, 287, 1985.

913 **White, M. A. and Bucci, L. R.,** Succinate effect on mouse swimming performance, *J Appl Sport Sci Res*, 2(3), 52, 1988

914 **Ariel, G. and Saville, W.,** Anabolic steroids: the physiological effects of placebos, *Med Sci Sports*, 4, 124, 1972

915 Regulations under the Federal Food, Drug and Cosmetic Act, Code of Federal Regulations, Part 133, Title 21 U S Department of Health, Education, and Welfare, Food and Drug Administration, 1985

916. **Cerretelli, P. and Marconi, C.,** L-Carnitine supplementation in humans The effects on physical performance, *Int J Sports Med* , 11(1), 1, 1990
917 **Desnuelle, C., Pellissier, J. F., de Barsy, T., and Serratrice, G.,** Intolerance to exercise caused by carnitine palmitoyltransferase deficiency, *Rev Neurol* , 146, 231, 1990.
918 **Broderick, T. L., Poirier, P., Tremblay, A., Catellier, C., and Nadeau, A.,** Effect of exogenous insulin on plasma free carnitine levels during exercise in normal man, *Can J Physiol Pharmacol* , 67, 1589, 1989
919 **Harris, R. C., Foster, C. V. L., and Hultman, E.,** Acetylcarnitine formation during intense muscular contraction in humans, *J Appl Physiol* , 63, 440, 1987
920 **Hiatt, W. R., Regensteiner, J. G., Wolfel, E. E., Ruff, L., and Brass, E. P.,** Carnitine and acylcarnitine metabolism during exercise in humans Dependence on skeletal muscle metabolic state, *J Clin Invest* , 84, 1167, 1989.
921 **Sahlin, K.,** Muscle carnitine metabolism during incremental dynamic exercise in humans, *Acta Physiol Scand.,* 138, 259, 1990
922 **Constantin-Teodosiu, D., Carlin, J. I., Cederblad, G., Harris, R. C., and Hultman, E.,** Acetyl group accumulation and pyruvate dehydrogenase activity in human muscle during incremental exercise, *Acta Physiol Scand* , 143, 367, 1991.
923. **Arenas, J., Ricoy, J. R., Encinas, A. R., Pola, P., Diddio, S., Zeviani, M., Didonato, S., and Corsi, M.,** Carnitine in muscle, serum and the urine of nonprofessional athletes: effects of physical exercise, training and L-carnitine administration, *Muscle Nerve*, 14, 598, 1991.
924 **Decombaz, J., Gmuender, B., Sierro, G., and Cerretelli, P.,** Muscle carnitine after strenuous endurance exercise, *J Appl Physiol* , 72, 423, 1992
925 **Suzuki, M., Kanaya, M., Muramutsu, S., and Takahashi, T.,** Effects of carnitine administration, fasting and exercise on urinary carnitine excretion in man, *J Nutr Sci Vitaminol* , 22, 169, 1976
926 **Dragan, G. J., Vasiliu, A., Georgescu, E., and Dumas, I.,** Studies concerning chronic and acute effects of L-carnitine on some biological parameters in elite athletes, *Physiologie,* 24, 23, 1987
927. **Dragan, A. M., Vasiliu, A., Eremia, N. M., and Georgescu, E.,** Studies concerning some acute biological changes after endovenous administration of 1 g L-carnitine in elite athletes, *Physiologie,* 24, 231, 1987
928. **Dragan, I. G., Vasiliu, A., Georgescu, E., and Eremia, N.,** Studies concerning chronic and acute effects of L-carnitine in elite athletes, *Physiologie,* 26, 111, 1989
929 **Vecchiet, L., Di Lisa, F., Pieralisi, G., Ripari, P., Menabo, R., Giamberardino, M. A., and Siliprandi, N.,** Influence of L-carnitine administration on maximal physical performance, *Eur J Appl. Physiol* , 61, 486, 1990
930 **Siliprandi, N., Di Lisa, F., Pieralisi, G., Pipari, P., Maccari, F., Menabo, R., Giamberardino, M. A., and Vecchiet, L.,** Metabolic changes induced by maximal exercise in human subjects following L-carnitine administration, *Biochim Biophys Acta,* 1034, 17, 1990.
931. **Gorostiaga, E. M., Maurer, C. A., and Eclache, J. P.,** Decrease in respiratory quotient during exercise following L-carnitine supplementation, *Int J Sports Med* , 10, 164, 1989
932 **Wyss, V., Ganzit, G. P., and Rienzi, A.,** Effects of L-carnitine administration on VO_2max and the aerobic-anaerobic threshold in normoxia and hypoxia, *Eur J Appl Physiol* , 60, 1, 1990
933 **Corbucci, G. G., Montanari, G., Mancinelli, G., and Diddio, S.,** Metabolic effects induced by L-carnitine and propionyl-L-carnitine in human hypoxic muscle tissue during exercise, *Int J Clin Pharmacol Res* , 10, 197, 1990
934 **Goa, K. L. and Brodgen, R. N.,** L-carnitine. A preliminary review of its pharmacokinetics, and its therapeutic use in ischaemic heart disease and primary and secondary carnitine deficiences in relationship to its role in fatty acid metabolism, *Drugs,* 34, 1, 1987

935 Cherchi, A., Lai, C., Onnis, E., Orani, E., Pirisi, R., Pisano, M. R., Soro, A., and
     Corsi, M., Propionyl carnitine in stable effort angina, *Cardiovasc Drugs Ther* , 4(2), 481,
     1990

936. Cacciatore, L., Cerio, R., Ciarimboli, M., Cocozza, M., Coto, V., DAlessandro, A.,
     DAlessandro, L., Grattarola, G., Imparato, L., and Lingetti, M., The therapeutic effect
     of L-carnitine in patients with exercise-induced stable angina: a controlled study, *Drugs
     Exp Clin. Res* , 17, 225, 1991

937. Brevetti, G., Perna, S., Sabba, C., Rossini, A., Scotto di Uccio, V., Berardi, E., and
     Godi, L., Superiority of L-propionylcarnitine vs. L-carnitine in improving walking capac-
     ity in patients with peripheral vascular disease: an acute, intravenous, double-blind, cross-
     over study, *Eur Heart J* , 13, 251, 1992

938 Kobayashi, A., Masumura, Y., and Yamazaki, N., L-carnitine treatment for congestive
     heart failure — experimental and clinical study, *Jpn Circ J* , 56, 86, 1992

939 Lagioia, R., Scrutinio, D., Mangini, S. G., Ricci, A., Mastropasqua, F., Valentini, G.,
     Ramunni, G., Totaro-Fila, G., and Rizzon, P., Propionyl-L-carnitine: a new compound
     in the metabolic approach to treatment of effort angina, *Int J Cardiol* , 34, 167, 1992.

940. Ahmad, S., Robertson, H. T., Golper, T. A., Wolfson, M., Kurtin, P., Katz, L. A.,
     Hirschberg, R., Nicora, R., Ashbrook, D. W., and Kopple, J. D., Multicenter trial of L-
     carnitine in maintenance hemodialysis patients II. Clinical and biochemical effects, *Kidney
     Int* , 38, 912, 1990

941. Lenaz, G., Ed., *Coenzyme Q Biochemistry. Bioenergetics and Clinical Applications of
     Ubiquinone,* John Wiley, Chichester, U.K., 1985.

942 Beyer, R. E., The role of coenzyme Q in endurance training-acquired resistance to free
     radical damage, in *Biomedical and Clinical Aspects of Coenzyme Q,* Vol 6, Folkers, K.,
     Yamagami, T., and Littarru, G. P , Eds , Elsevier, Amsterdam, 1991, 501

943 Ernster, L. and Beyer, R. E., Antioxidant functions of coenzyme Q: some biochemical
     and pathophysiological implications, in *Biomedical and Clinical Aspects of Coenzyme Q,*
     Vol 6, Folkers, K , Yamagami, T , and Littarru, G P., Eds , Elsevier, Amsterdam,
     1991, 45.

944. Lenaz, G., Barnabei, O., Rabbi, A., and Battino, M., Eds., *Highlights in Ubiquinone
     Research,* Taylor & Francis, London, 1990.

945 Folkers, K. and Yamamura, Y., Eds., *Biomedical and Clinical Aspects of Coenzyme Q,*
     Vol. 5, Elsevier, Amsterdam, 1986.

946 Folkers, K., Yamagami, T., and Littarru, G. P., *Biomedical and Clinical Aspects* of
     Coenzyme Q, Vol 6, Elsevier, Amsterdam, 1991.

947. Lenaz, G., Fato, R., Castelluccio, C., Batino, M., Cavazzoni, M., Rauchova, H., and
     Castelli, G. P., Coenzyme Q saturation kinetics of mitochondrial enzymes: theory, experi-
     mental aspects and biomedical implications, in *Biomedical and Clinical Aspects of Coen-
     zyme Q,* Vol 6, Folkers, K., Yamagami, T , and Littarru, G. P., Eds., Elsevier, Amsterdam,
     1991, 11

948 Karlsson, J., Diamant, B., Theorell, H., and Folkers, K., Skeletal muscle coenzyme Q_{10}
     in healthy man and selected patient groups, in *Biomedical and Clinical Aspects of Coen-
     zyme Q,* Vol 6, Folkers, K , Yamagami, T , and Littarru, G. P., Eds., Elsevier, Amsterdam,
     1991, 191

949. Karlsson, J., Diamant, B., Folkers, K., Edlund, P.-O., Lund, B., and Theorell, H.,
     Skeletal muscle and blood CoQ_{10} in health and disease, in *Highlights in Ubiquinone
     Research,* Lenaz, G., Barnabei, O , Rabbi, A., and Battino, M., Eds , Taylor & Francis,
     London, 1990, 288

950 Guerra, G. P., Ballardini, E., Lippa, S., Oradei, A., and Littarru, G. P., Effetto della
     somministrazione di Ubidecarenone nel consume massimo di ossigeno e sulla performance
     fisica in un gruppo di giovani ciclisti, *Medicina dello Sport,* 40, 359, 1987

951 Karlsson, J., Heart and skeletal muscle ubiquinone (CoQ_{10}) as a protective agent against
     radical formation in man, in *Advances in Myochemistry,* Benzi, G , Ed., John Libbey
     Eurotext, London, 1987, 305.

952 **Littarru, G. P., Lippa, S., Oradei, A., Aureli, V., and Serino, F.,** Factors affecting blood and tissue levels of CoQ_{10} in vitro and in vivo studies, in *Highlights in Ubiquinone Research,* Lenaz, G , Barnabei, O., Rabbi, A., and Battino, M., Eds., Taylor & Francis, London, 1990, 220

953 **Vanfraechem, J. and Folkers, K.,** Coenzyme Q_{10} and physical performance, in *Biomedical and Clinical Aspects of Coenzyme Q,* Vol 3, Folkers, K and Yamamura, Y., Eds , Elsevier, Amsterdam, 1981, 235

954 **Yamabe, H. and Fukuzaki, H.,** The beneficial effect of coenzyme Q_{10} on the impaired aerobic function in middle aged women without organic disease, in *Biomedical and Clinical Aspects of Coenzyme Q,* Vol 6, Folkers, K., Yamagami, T., and Littarru, G P., Eds., Elsevier, Amsterdam, 1991, 535.

955. **Cerioli, G., Tirelli, G., and Musiani, L.,** Effect of CoQ_{10} on the metabolic response to work, in *Biomedical and Clinical Aspects of Coenzyme Q,* Vol. 6, Folkers, K , Yamagami, T , and Littarru, G. P , Eds., Elsevier, Amsterdam, 1991, 521

956 **Morishita, R., Chen, W.-L., and Eguchi, T.,** Effects of Ubiquinone-10 on lipid metabolism in patients with hyperlipidemia,*Vitamins,* 57, 665, 1983

957 **Zeppilli, P., Merlino, B., de Luca, A., Palmieri, V., Santini, C., Vannicelli, R., la Rosa Gangi, M., Caccese, R., Cameli, S., Servidei, S., Ricci, E., Silvestri, G., Lippa, S., Oradei, A., and Littaru, G. P.,** Influence of coenzyme Q_{10} on physicl work capacity in athletes, sedentary people and patients with mitochondrial disease, in *Biomedical and Clinical Aspects of Coenzyme Q,* Vol. 6, Folkers, K., Yamagami, T., and Littarru, G P , Eds , Elsevier, Amsterdam, 1991, 541

958 **Wyss, V., Lubich, T., Ganzit, G. P., Cesaretti, D., Fiorella, P. L., Dei Rocini, C., Bargossi, A. M., Battistoni, R., Lippi, A., Grossi, G., Sprovieri, G., and Battino, M.,** Remarks on prolonged ubiquinone administration in physical exercise, in *Highlights in Ubiquinone Research,* Lenaz, G , Barnabei, O , Rabbi, A , and Battino, M., Eds , Taylor & Francis, London, 1990, 303.

959 **Fiorella, P. L., Bargossi, A. M., Grossi, G., Motta, R., Senaldi, R., Battino, M., Sassi, S., Sprovieri, G., and Lubich, T.,** Metabolic effects of coenzyme Q_{10} treatment in high level athletes, in *Biomedical and Clinical Aspects of Coenzyme Q,* Vol 6, Folkers, K., Yamagami, T , and Littarru, G. P., Eds , Elsevier, Amsterdam, 1991, 513

960 **Amadio, E., Palermo, R., Peloni, G., and Littarru, G. P.,** Effect of CoQ_{10} administration on VO_2max and diastolic function in athletes, in *Biomedical and Clinical Aspects of Coenzyme Q,* Vol 6, Folkers, K , Yamagami, T., and Littarru, G., P , Eds., Elsevier, Amsterdam, 1991, 525

961. **Rossi, E., Lombardo, A., Testa, M., Lippa, S., Oradei, A., Littarru, G. P., Lucente, M., Coppola, E., and Manzoli, U.,** Coenzyme Q_{10} in ischaemic cardiopathy, in *Biomedical and Clinical Aspects of Coenzyme Q,* Vol 6, Folkers, K., Yamagami, T , and Littarru, G P , Eds., Elsevier, Amsterdam, 1991, 321

962. **Wilson, M. F., Frishman, W. H., Giles, T., Sethi, G., Greenberg, S. M., and Brackett, D. J.,** Coenzyme Q_{10} therapy and exercise duration in stable angina, in *Biomedical and Clinical Aspects of Coenzyme Q,* Vol 6, Folkers, K , Yamagami, T , and Littarru, G P , Eds , Elsevier, Amsterdam, 1991, 339

963 **Greenberg, S. M. and Frishman, W. H.,** Coenzyme Q_{10}: a new drug for myocardial ischemia, *Med Clin N Am ,* 72, 243, 1988

INDEX

A

Acetyl carnitine, 47
Acetylcholine, 61
Acetyl groups, 47
Acidosis, 13, 41
Acylcarnitines, 47, 48
Acyl transferase, 47
Adenine, 62
Adenosine, 61, 62
Adenosine triphosphate (ATP), 97
  ammonia and, 70
  arginine and, 70
  aspartate salts and, 45
  carnitine and, 47, 49
  coenzyme Q_{10} and, 53, 54
  creatine and, 57
  glutamate and, 72
  intracellular, 31
  loss of, 70
  muscle, 30
  nucleic acids and, 61
  ornithine and, 75
  production of, 18, 37, 54
  vitamin B and, 30, 31
  vitamin C and, 37
S-Adenosyl methionine (SAM), 58, 61
Adipose tissue, 18
Alanine, 18
Albumin, 76
Alcohol, 4, 83
Aldolase, 41
Alkaline loading, 41, 42
Alkalinizers, 41–42, see also specific types
Alkalosis, 41, 42
Allithiamines, 31, see also specific types
Aminoacetic acid, see Glycine
Amino acids, 9, 14, 16, 18, 69–78, 91, 97,
    105, see also specific types
  branched-chain, 25, 47, 72, 77
  chromium and, 68
  combination of with other nutrients, 79
  dicarboxylic, 45
  guidelines for, 71
  metabolism of, 24, 63
  minerals and, 63
  mixtures of, 16
  summary of ergogenic properties of, 77–78
  supplementation of, 17
  vitamin B and, 24, 25

p-Aminobenzoic acid (PABA), 30
Ammonia, 46, 47, 56
  detoxification of, 70–71
  intracellular, 72
  ornithine and, 75
  plasma, 71, 72
Ammonium chloride, 64
Amphetamines, 2, 5, see also specific types
Anabolic steroids, 2–4, 15, 18, 101, 102, see
    also specific types
  chromium and, 68
  ferulates and, 91
  vitamin B_{12} and, 27
Analgesics, 5, see also specific types
Androgenic steroids, 2, see also specific types
Anemia, 65
Anesthetics, 5, see also specific types
Angina, 62
Animal research, 102
Antihistamines, 2, see also specific types
Antioxidant enzymes, 43, 44, see also spe-
    cific types
Antioxidants, 34, 36–38, 42–45, see also spe-
    cific types
  ferulic acid as, 90
  guidelines for, 44–45, 106
  human studies on, 43–44
  pollen and, 95
  selenium as, 67, 68
Apolipoprotein A, 31
Arachidonic acid, 19
Archery, 32
Arginine, 57, 69–73, 77, 78
  combination of with other nutrients, 79
  glycine and, 74
  growth hormone and, 69–70
  guidelines for, 71
  ornithine and, 75
Arginine aspartate, 69–71
Arginine glutamate, 72
Arginine infusion test, 69
Arginineornithine, 71
Arginine pyroglutamate, 70, 78
Ascorbic acid, see Vitamin C
Ascorbyl palmitate, 34, 97
Aspartate, 45, 77
Aspartate salts, 45–47, 71, 78
Aspartic acid, 45, 71, 75
Astrand (classical) regimen, 9–10
ATP, see Adenosine triphosphate

NOTES